AF564764

BODY IMAGE, HUMAN REPRODUCTION AND BIRTH CONTROL

A TRIBAL PERSPECTIVE

BODY IMAGE HUMAN REPRODUCTION AND BIRTH CONTROL

A TRIBAL PERSPECTIVE

By

Dr. ROBIN D. TRIBHUWAN
M.A., M.Sc. P.G.D.M., Ph.D.

&

Dr. BENAZIR D. PATIL
M.A., Ph.D.

DISCOVERY PUBLISHING HOUSE PVT. LTD.
NEW DELHI-110 002

First Published-2009

ISBN 978-81-8356-388-8

Published by:

DISCOVERY PUBLISHING HOUSE PVT. LTD.
4831/24, Ansari Road, Prahlad Street
Darya Ganj, New Delhi-110002 (India)
Phone: 23279245 • Fax: 91-11-23253475
E-mail: dphbooks@rediffmail.com
dphtemp@indiatimes.com
web: www.discoverypublishinghouse.com

Printed at:

Sachin Printers
Delhi

Foreword

Majority of tribal people in India live on the mountains and hills, in the valleys and forests away from the mainstream population. Monographs on tribal communities by anthropologists and sociologists have revealed that the tribals live aloof from the non-tribal settlements. Tribal hamlets are usually away from the non-tribal villages. In Maharashtra, some of the popular names for tribal hamlets are Phali, among the Bhils; Pada, among the Warlis; Wadi, among the Thakars and Katkaris; and Pod, among the Kolams. Members of every tribe living within a hamlet have always shown greater signs of solidarity, when it comes to sharing of common cultural beliefs.

Every tribe has its own cultural identity and dialect; hence, it is different from the other group. Tribe specific cultural traits and dialects have contributed in preserving common cultural beliefs and practices within a tribe. Health is an aspect of culture; hence all beliefs and practices regarding health, disease, body image, reproduction, healing etc develop from indigenous cultures. I have hardly read and heard of studies dealing with tribal perceptions of relativity between body image, human reproduction and birth control.

Dr. Robin Tribhuwan, an eminent anthropologist and development expert along with Dr. Benazir Patil, a policy specialist in health and social development have sparked an interest of theoretical as well as practical significance for social, health and medical scientists to conduct further research region or tribe-wise in the above mentioned areas.

I wish the authors and this venture a success.

Dr. Vijay Kumar Gavit
Minister
Tribal Development
Government of Maharashtra, Mantralaya
Mumbai – 400 032

Preface

Tribals in India have been living on the mountains, the hills and in the forests and valleys in isolation for ages. These geographical areas were not easily accessible. As a result tribals remained cut off from the outside world and led their lives in isolation. They have lived very close to the nature and have been meeting their sustainable needs from the local environment, which include food, shelter and medicine. Infact several tribes have developed a body of folk mythology, perceptions of body image, reproduction, ethno physiology, ethno anatomy etc. from what they have observed for ages, among the animal and plant world around them. Infact a number tribes have developed ritual relationship with the flora and fauna around them. For a long time they have been facing the forces of nature unitedly, following their indigenous wisdom and knowledge.

This body of knowledge and indigenous wisdom was passed on from one generation to another by word of mouth, through oral tradition. From the tribal perspective, the rationale, the logic, the beliefs and practices associated with their indigenous wisdom makes sense. However, the emic (insider's) views of tribals about human body, reproduction, medicine, disease, health, birth control etc. differ from the allopathic or scientific – the etic (outsider's) views.

Interestingly, the health care providers in the primary health sector have adopted the allopathic or scientific view to provide health care and education to the tribals. This gives no scope to the traditional wisdom and knowledge of tribals regarding disease, health, medicine, body image etc. But, the fact remains that the 750 tribes existing in this country are influenced and practice their traditional medicine, because it makes sense to them.

This study has unveiled the traditional wisdom and knowledge of five tribes namely: Thakars, Santhals, Gonds, Mavchis and Ao Nagas about their perceptions regarding body image, human reproduction and birth control. The basic objective of the book is to demonstrate that despite of 57 years of independence and the influence of modernisation, India has several tribes who still respect, believe and practice their traditional medicine. We have suggested the need to scientifically study and analyse these practices so as to make them safe, secured, accessible and scientifically valid to promote its use for the tribals.

Infact Dr. Samba, WHO's Regional Director for Africa, comments that if 80 per cent of the people in Africa really use traditional medicine, "we must move quickly to evaluate its safety, efficacy, quality and standardisation—to protect our heritage and preserve our traditional knowledge". He further comments that we must also institutionalise and integrate it into our national health system.

We hope that Dr. Samba's message reaches the primary health centres and sub-centres of India, that work in Tribal areas. This study is just a drop in an ocean, but it will certainly create interest among social, health and medical scientists to take up multi-disciplinary studies to explore scientifically into the area of tribal medicine, health, disease, body image, human reproduction and birth control.

Dr. Robin D. Tribhuwan
Dr. Benazir D. Patil

Contents

1

Medicine, Birth Control and Contraceptive Practices

Traditional and Modern Perspective

INTRODUCTION

Disease in some or the other form has been a fundamental problem of every society and every known society has developed ways, means and methods of coping with disease, thereby creating a system of medicine. Thus, even before the advent of modern medicine, people all over the world had developed culture specific beliefs and practices regarding health and disease.

It is to such beliefs and practices which are products of indigenous cultural development and are not explicitly derived from the conceptual framework of modern medicine that the term. "ethno-medicine," is applied to. Ever since the dawn of his turbulent history man has evolved several ways of coping with illness. All ancient civilisations have thus developed their own medical system which not only reflect certain philosophies but also appears to be influenced by the then existing social beliefs and practices.

Literature on medicine and various medical systems known to mankind is available on biological and cultural aspects of health and disease. Anthropological interest in medicine stems from the fact that health and disease though biological in nature are defined and interpreted culturally as they are related to people's social belief systems. Infact, medical Anthropologists are of the view that health is an integral aspect of culture.

The theoretical concern of medical anthropology is made explicit by Lieban, who stated that, "medical Anthropology encompasses the study of medical phenomena as they are influenced by social and cultural features and social and cultural phenomena as they are illuminated by their medical aspects." At the more practical level the study of medically related beliefs and practices assumes significance in developing and implementing culturally acceptable health care services and health education programmes.

India is an Anthropological Laboratory having different cultures, ethnic groups, languages, medical systems and diverse belief systems deeply rooted in their respective cultures. Every cultural group in India has beliefs and practices regarding:

- Origin and cause of disease and illness
- Classification of disease
- Body image, ethno-anatomy and ethno-physiology
- Functions of various biological systems in the body
- Impact of hot, cold and lukewarm food, water, fluids, air etc on the various bodily systems and organs
- Maternal and child health care
- Body, mind and soul
- Birth control and contraception

These beliefs and practices are observed in daily life of people of a given culture. An orthodox Hindu will never drink coffee immediately after he has had "Lassi", for he fears the impact of hot (Coffee) and cold (lassi) elements that might disturb his bodily equilibrium. A tribal woman (Thakars) will net feed her child with colostrum milk (naska dudh) as she fears that it may lead to indigestion as it is believed to be spoilt milk.

On one hand, as social scientists we observe the above health behaviours in various societies in India, but on the other hand we also see that the rationale of primary health care and health education is primarily based on allopathic philosophy. This no doubt contradicts which the indigenous peoples' health beliefs and practices. Infact the number of health care providers and health educators in the health departments of our country both in urban and rural areas are people from allopathy or modern medicine, which tend to give less or no importance to peoples' health beliefs and practices.

This book primarily throws light on tribal beliefs and practices regarding body image, human reproduction process, traditional birth control practices and contraception in the larger context of ethno medicine, reproductive health and maternal and child health care beliefs and practices. The book is written to create awareness among health, medical and social scientists including the health care providers, that it is necessary to understand the rationale, the scientific base and optimism in tribal ethno-medical beliefs and practices regarding body image and birth control practices. Before getting into the medical world of tribals, at this juncture it is necessary to understand the concept of medicine, medical systems, global and Indian policies regarding contraception etc.

(a) The Institution of Medicine

Medicine is the science and art of maintaining and restoring human health through the study, diagnosis and treatment of patients. The term is derived from the Latin *ars medicina* meaning *the art of healing.*

The modern practice of medicine occurs at the many interfaces between *the art of healing* and various sciences. Medicine is directly connected to the health sciences and biomedicine. Broadly speaking, the term 'Medicine' today refers to the fields of clinical medicine, medical research and surgery, thereby covering the challenges of disease and injury.

The earliest type of medicine in most cultures was the use of empirical natural resources like plants (herbalism), animal parts and minerals. In all societies, including Western ones, there were also religious, ritual and magical resources. In aboriginal societies, there is a large scope of *medical systems* related to religious thinking, cultural experience, and natural resources. The religious ones more known are: animism (the notion of inanimate objects having spirits); spiritualism (here meaning an appeal to gods or communion with ancestor spirits); shamanism (the vesting of an individual with mystic powers); and divination (the supposed obtaining of truth by magic means). The field of medical anthropology studies the various medical systems and their interaction with society, while prehistoric addresses diagnosis and treatment in prehistoric times.

The practice of medicine developed gradually in ancient Egypt, Babylonia, India, China, Greece, Persia, the Islamic world, medieval Europe and early modern period in Persia (Rhazes and Avicenna), Spain (Abulcasis and Avenzoar), Syria/Egypt (Ibn al-Nafis, 13th century), Italy (Gabriele Falloppio, 16th century), England (William Harvey, 17th century). Medicine as it is now practiced largely developed during the 19th and 20th centuries in Germany (Rudolf Virchow, Wilhelm Conrad Röntgen, Robert Koch), Austria (Karl Landsteiner, Otto Loewi), United Kingdom (Edward Jenner, Alexander Fleming, Joseph Lister, Francis Crick), New Zealand (Maurice Wilkins), Australia (Howard Floery, Frank Macfarlane Burnet), Russia (Nikolai Korotkov), United States (William Williams Keen, Harvey Cushing, William Coley, James D. Watson), Italy (Salvador Luria), Switzerland (Alexandre Yersin), Japan (Kitasato Shibasaburo), and France (Jean-Martin Charcot, Claude Bernard, Louis Pasteur, Paul Broca and others). The new "scientific" or "experimental" medicine (where results are testable and repeatable) replaced early Western traditions of medicine, based on herbalism, the Greek "four humours" and other pre-modern theories.

The Sumerian god Ningizzida was the patron of medicine. In the image he is accompanied by two gryphons. It is the oldest known image of snakes coiling around an axial rod, dating from before 2000 BCE. A similar image with two snakes coiling around a rod is called the Caduceus and, although historically inappropriate, appears in the logo/emblem of a significant number of private (rather than professional or academic) medical practices.

The focal points of development of clinical medicine shifted to the United Kingdom and the USA by the early 1900s (Canadian-born) Sir William Osler, Harvey Cushing). Possibly the major shift in medical thinking was the gradual rejection, especially during the Black Death in the 14th and 15th centuries, of what may be called the 'traditional authority' approach to science and medicine. This was the notion that because some prominent person in the past said something must be so, then that was the way it was, and anything one observed to the contrary was an anomaly (which was paralleled by a similar shift in European society in general—see Copernicus's rejection of Ptolemy's theories on astronomy). Physicians like Ibn al-Nafis and Vesalius led the way in improving upon or indeed rejecting the theories of great authorities from the past (such as Hippocrates, Galen and Avicenna), many of whose theories were in time discredited. Such new attitudes were made possible in Europe by the weakening of the Roman Catholic Church's power in society, especially in the Republic of Venice.

Evidence-based medicine is a recent movement to establish the most effective algorithms of practice (ways of doing things) through the use of the scientific method and modern global information science by collating all the evidence and developing standard protocols which are then disseminated to healthcare providers. One problem with this 'best practice' approach is that it could be seen to stifle novel approaches to treatment.

The practice of medicine combines both science as the evidence base and art in the application of this medical knowledge in combination with intuition and clinical judgment to determine the treatment plan for each patient.

According to Tribhuwan Robin (1998:9), the institution of medicine can be analysed from two angles namely the biomedical and socio-cultural.

(a) *Bio-medical:* This angle of medicine interprets disease on the lines of germ theory.

b) *Socio-cultural:* This aspect associates the origin and cause of disease to intervention of spiritual, cosmic, ancestral, supernatural and socio-pathogenic agents/ forces.

In case of tribals the second aspect is important. Understanding their ethno-medical beliefs and practices regarding health and disease becomes significant from the point of view of delivering health care and health educational services to them. It is necessary at this juncture to know the concept of traditional medicine and the various types of medical systems. Given below are few examples of medical systems.

(b) Traditional Medicine and Medical Systems

Traditional Medicine

The term *traditional medicine (Indigenous medicine or folk medicine)* describes medical knowledge systems, which developed over centuries within various societies before the era of modern medicine; traditional medicines include practices such as herbal medicine, Ayurvedic medicine, Unani medicine, Acupuncture, Siddha Medicine, traditional Chinese medicine, South African Muṭi, Yoruba Ifá, as well as other medical knowledge and practices all over the globe.

WHO defines traditional medicine as: the health practices, approaches, knowledge and beliefs incorporating plant, animal and mineral based medicines, spiritual therapies, manual techniques and exercises, applied singularly or in combination to treat, diagnose and prevent illnesses or maintain well-being.

Countries in Africa, Asia and Latin America use traditional medicine to help meet some of their primary health care needs. For example, in Africa, up to 80 per cent of the population uses traditional medicine for primary health care. The WHO, however, also notes that its use is spreading in popularity in industrialised countries. For example, in the United States, 158 million adults use complementary medicine (a field which incorporates traditional medicine but is broader in scope).

The WHO also notes, though, that "inappropriate use of traditional medicines or practices can have negative or dangerous effects" and that "further research is needed to ascertain the efficacy and safety" of several of the practices and medicinal plants used by traditional medicine systems.

Core disciplines which study traditional medicine include ethno-medicine, ethno-botany, and medical anthropology. Traditional medicine is full of real experiences, observations and fancy formulae reflecting a combination of inspiration, facts and results. However, some concepts are beyond the realm of rational and experimental analysis in contemporary terms. In the words of Caraka—one of the most eminent Ayurvedic scholars of ancient India—*"there is very little that can be obtained by direct proof. The province beyond direct experimental evidence is vast. This can be obtained by inference, rational thinking and advices of teachers and other experts in the field"*.

(i) Ayurveda—the Medicinal System from Ancient India

In ancient context, India has been blessed with several perspectives which talk about not just diseases and illnesses but an overall well-being of human beings. Ayurveda is a broad based science of life developed with 2 fold objectives—to preserve the health of a healthy individual and to relieve the disease of the ailing.

Virtually every country has a system of traditional medicines possessing a unique configuration designed to be compatible with its own future and meeting the needs of its own populations. Therefore Ayurvedic thoughts and methods have had a deep impact in the life style of the people of India.

According to Ayurveda, life is a combination of Body, Senses, Spirit, Soul and Mind. Thus health means the healthy state of all these components. The *concepts in treatment.*

The theory of *Panchamahabuta* and the theory of *Tri Dosha* are the basis of Ayurveda:

1. According to the theory of *Panchamahabhuta*, every creation is a combination of 5 subtle elements – Space (*Akasha*), Air (Vayu), Fire (*Agni*), Water (Jala) and Earth (*Prithvi*).
2. The theory of *Tri Dosha* is a deeper biological application of the concept of *Panchamahabhuta. Tri Dosha* or the three humors are *Vata, Pitta*, and *Kapha*.

Vata is characterized by the predominance of *Vayu* and *Akasa*. *Pitta* is formed by the action of *Agni* and *Kapha* formed by the *Jala* and *Prithvi*. These are called as doshas because they have the the tendency to get vitiated and to vitiate other elements of the body. They are considered as *dhatus* as they help to upload the body.

The equilibrium of the three *doshas* keeps the body healthy. When this equilibrium is lost body becomes diseases. To maintain the equilibrium and to reestablish the disturbed equilibrium, substance having similar properties or opposite properties are used accordingly to the condition. If *Vata Dosha* is increased in a body, this may cause *Vata* diseases. To cure this, the increased *Vata* must be normalised. For this substances and habits having properties opposite to that of *Vata* are practiced. If *Vata Dosha* is decreased it will also disturb the equilibrium. This will cause diseases, which are cured by increasing *Vata* in the body. For that the substances and habits which increase *Vata* are used. This constitutes the basic principle of Ayurvedic treatments.

Apart from the three humours, Ayurveda explain 7 *dhatus*. These are related with the normal function of the body. These can be compared to the tissues of modern science. The 7 *dhatus* are:

1. *Rasa* (Plasma)
2. *Rakta* (Blood)
3. *Mamsa* (Muscles)
4. *Medas* (Fat)
5. *Asthi* (Bone)
6. *Majja* (Marrow)
7. *Sukra* (Reproductive elements)

The vitiation of the three humours will vitiate *dhatus* and the vitiation will manifest as diseases. Thus the *dhatus* can be considered as the materialised forms of the three *Dosha*. Thus the treatment in Ayurveda can concluded as the processing of maintaining equilibrium of these factors.

(ii) Unani Medicine—Greco-Arabic

It is used to refer to ***Graeco-Arabic*** or ***Unani*** medicine, also called "Unani-tibb", based on the teachings of Hippocrates, Galen, and Avicenna, and based on the four humours Phlegm (*Balgham*), Blood (*Dam*), Yellow bile (*Safra*) and Black bile (*Sauda* — it seems to mean hard substance and black material).

Though the threads which comprise Unani healing can be traced all the way back to Claudius Galenus of Pergamum, who lived in the second century of the Christian Era, the basic knowledge of Unani medicine as a healing system was developed by Hakim Ibn Sina (known as Avicenna in the west) in his medicial encyclopaedia *The Canon of Medicine*. The time of origin is thus dated at *circa* 1025 AD, when Avicenna wrote *The Canon of Medicine* in Persia. While he was primarily influenced by Greek and Islamic medicine, he was also influenced by the Indian medical teachings of *Sushruta* and *Charaka*.

As an alternative medicine, Unani has found favour in Asia, especially India. In India, Unani practitioners can practice as qualified doctors, as the Indian government approves their practice. Unani medicine is very close to Ayurveda. Both are based on theory of the presence of the elements (in Unani, they are considered to be fire, water, earth and air) in the human body. (The elements, attributed to the philosopher Empedocles, determined the way of thinking in mediaeval Europe.) According to followers of Unani medicine, these elements are present in different fluids and their balance leads to health and their imbalance leads to illness.

All these elaborations were built on the basic Hippocratic theory of the "Four Humours". The theory postulates the presence in the human body of blood, phlegm, yellow bile and black bile. Each person's unique mixture of these substances determines his temperament: a predominance of blood gives a sanguine temperament; a predominance of phlegm makes one phlegmatic; yellow bile, bilious (or choleric); and black bile, melancholic. As long as these humours are in balance, the human system is healthy; it is imbalance which can result in disease.

Most medicines and remedies (often common herbs and foods) used in Unani are also used in Ayurveda. While Unani was influenced by Islam, Ayurveda is associated with Vedic culture.

The base used in Unani medicine is often honey. Honey is considered by some to have healing properties and hence is used in food and medicines practiced in the Islamic world. Real pearls and metal are also used in the making of Unani medicine based on the kind of ailment it is aimed to heal.

(iii) Siddha System

The Siddha system of medicine is a form of south Indian traditional medicine and part of the trio Indian medicines—Ayurveda, Siddha and Unani. This system of medicine was popular in ancient India, even 2000 years before Christ due to the antiquity of this medical system. The Siddha system of medicine is believed to be the oldest medical system in the universe. The system is believed to be developed by the Siddhars, the ancient supernatural spiritual saints of India and the Siddha system is believed to be handed over to the Siddhar by the Hindu God—Lord Shiva and Goddess Parvathi. So are the Siddhars, the followers of Lord Shiva (*saivam*).

According to the scriptures, there were 18 principal Siddhars. Of these 18, saint Agasthiyar is believed to be the father of Siddha Medicine. There is a controversy that exists in this regard as some people claim, Siddhar Theraiyyar (One of the 18 Siddhars) as the Father of Siddha Medicine.

Siddhars were of the concept that a healthy soul can only be developed through a healthy body. So they developed methods and medication that are believed to strengthen their physical body and thereby their souls. They practiced intense yogic practices, including years of fasting and meditation and believed to have achieved supernatural powers and gained the supreme wisdom and overall immortality.

Through this spiritually attained supreme knowledge, they wrote scriptures on all aspects of life, from arts to science and truth of life to miracle cure for diseases. The Siddhars wrote their knowledge in palm leaf manuscripts, fragments of which were found in different parts of South India. It is believed that some families may possess more fragments, but keep them solely for their own use.

From these manuscripts, the Siddha System of medicine developed into a part of Indian medical science. Today there are recognised Siddha Medical Colleges, run under the government universities where Siddha medicine is taught. Siddha medicine, like ayurveda, categories diseases into *Vata*, *Pitta* and *Kapha*.

(iv) Naturopathic Medicine

Naturopathic medicine (also known as Naturopathy) is a complementary and alternative medicine which emphasises the ability of the body to heal and maintain itself, which practitioners believe is innate. Naturopathic practice may include different modalities such as abstinence, acupuncture, colonic irrigation, counselling, chiropractic, diet, exercise, herbalism, homoeopathy, hydrotherapy, environmental medicine, manual therapy, orthomolecular medicine and relaxation. Practitioners emphasise a holistic approach to patient care, and may recommend patients use evidence-based medicine alongside their treatments. Naturopathy has its origins in a variety of world medicine practices, including the Ayurveda of India and Nature Cure of Europe. It is practiced in many countries but subject to different standards of regulation and levels of acceptance.

Naturopathic practitioners prefer not to use invasive surgery, or most synthetic drugs, preferring natural remedies, for instance relatively unprocessed or whole medications, such as herbs and foods. Practitioners from accredited schools are trained to use diagnostic tests such as imaging and blood tests before deciding upon the full course of treatment. If the patient does not respond to these treatments, they are often referred to physicians who utilise standard medical care to treat the disease or condition.

Naturopathic medicine went into decline, along with most other natural health professions, after the 1930s, with the discovery of penicillin and advent of synthetic drugs such as antibiotics and corticosteroids. In the post-war era, Lust's death, conflict between various schools of natural medicine (homoeopathy, eclectics, physio-medicalism, herbalism, naturopathy, etc.), and the rise of medical technology were all contributing factors. In 1910, when the Carnegie Foundation for the Advancement of Teaching published the Flexner Report which criticised many aspects of medical education in various institutions (natural and conventional), it was mostly seen as an attack on low-quality natural medicine education. It caused many such programmes to shut down and contributed to the popularity of conventional medicine.

Naturopathic medicine never completely ceased to exist, however, as there were always a few states in which licensing laws existed—though at one point there were virtually no schools. One of the most visible steps towards the profession's modern renewal was the opening in 1956 of the National College of Naturopathic Medicine in Portland, Oregon. This was the first of the modern naturopathic medical schools offering four-year naturopathic medical training wi h the intention of integrating science with naturopathic principles and practice.

(v) Islamic Medicine

The first Muslim physician is believed to have been Muhammad himself, as a significant number of hadiths concerning medicine are attributed to him. Several Sahaba are said to have been successfully treated of certain diseases by following the medical advice of Muhammad. The three methods of healing known to have been mentioned by him were honey, cupping, and cauterisation, though he was generally opposed to the use of cauterisation unless it "suits the ailment." According to Ibn Hajar al-Asqalani, Muhammad disliked this method due to it causing "pain and menace to a patient" since there was no anaesthesia in his time. Muhammad also appears to have been the first to suggest the contagious nature of leprosy, mange and sexually transmitted disease; and that there is always a cause and a cure for every disease, according to several hadiths in the Sahih al-Bukhari, Sunan Abi Dawood and Al-Muwatta attributed to Muhammad, such as:

"There is no disease that Allah has created, except that He also has created its treatment."

"Make use of medical treatment, for Allah has not made a disease without appointing a remedy for it, with the exception of one disease, namely old age."

"Allah has sent down both the disease and the cure, and He has appointed a cure for every disease, so treat yourselves medically."

"The one who sent down the disease sent down the remedy."

The belief that there is a cure for every disease encouraged early Muslims to engage in biomedical research and seek out a cure for every disease known to them. Many early authors of Islamic medicine, however, were usually clerics rather than physicians, and were known to have advocated the traditional medical practices of prophet Muhammad's time, such as those mentioned in the Qur'an and Hadith. For instance, therapy did not require a patient to undergo any surgical procedures at the time.

From the 9th century, Hunayn ibn Ishaq translated a number of Galen's works into the Arabic language, followed by translations of the *Sushruta Samhita*, *Charaka Samhita* and Middle Persian works from Gundishapur. Muslim physicians soon began making many of their own significant advances and contributions to medicine, including the fields of allergology, anatomy, bacteriology, botany, dentistry, embryology, environmentalism, etiology, immunology, microbiology, obstetrics, ophthalmology, pathology, paediatrics, perinatology, physiology, psychiatry, psychology, pulsology and sphygmology, surgery, therapy, urology, zoology, and the pharmaceutical sciences such as pharmacy and pharmacology, among others.

Medicine was a central part of mediaeval Islamic culture. Responding to circumstances of time and place, Islamic physicians and scholars developed a large and complex medical literature exploring and synthesising the theory and practice of medicine. Islamic medicine was initially built on tradition, chiefly the theoretical and practical knowledge developed in Arabia, Persia, Greece, Rome, and India. Galen and Hippocrates were pre-eminent authorities, as well as the Indian physicians Sushruta and Charaka, and the Hellenistic scholars in Alexandria. Islamic scholars translated their voluminous writings from Greek and Sanskrit into Arabic and then produced new medical knowledge based on those texts. In order to make the Greek and Indian traditions more accessible, understandable, and teachable, Islamic scholars ordered and made more systematic the vast and sometimes inconsistent Greco-Roman and Indian medical knowledge by writing encyclopaedias and summaries. It was through Arabic translations that the West learned of Hellenic medicine, including the works of Galen and Hippocrates. Of equal if not of greater influence in Western Europe were systematic and comprehensive works such as Avicenna's *The Canon of Medicine*, which were translated into Latin and then disseminated in manuscript and printed form throughout Europe. During the fifteenth and sixteenth centuries alone, *The Canon of Medicine* was published more than thirty-five times.

In etiology and epidemiology, Muslim physicians were responsible for the discovery of infectious disease and the immune system, advances in pathology, and early hypotheses related to bacteriology and microbiology. Their discovery of contagious disease in particular is considered revolutionary and is one of the most important discoveries in medicine. The earliest ideas on contagion can be traced back to several hadiths attributed to Muhammad in the 7th century, who is said to have understood the contagious nature of leprosy, mange, and sexually transmitted disease. These early ideas on contagion arose from the generally sympathetic attitude of Muslim physicians towards lepers (who were often seen in a negative light in other ancient and mediaeval societies) which can be traced back through hadiths attributed to Muhammad and to the following advice given in the Qur'an:

"There is no fault in the blind, and there is no fault in the lame, and there is no fault in the sick."

This eventually led to the theory of contagious disease, which was fully understood by Avicenna in the 11th century. By then, the pathology of contagion had been fully understood, and as a result, hospitals were created with separate wards for specific illnesses, so that people with contagious diseases could be kept away from other patients who do not have any contagious diseases. In *The Canon of Medicine* (1020), Avicenna discovered the contagious nature of infectious diseases such as phthisis and tuberculosis, the distribution of diseases by water and soil, and fully understood the contagious nature of sexually transmitted diseases. In epidemiology, he introduced the method of quarantine as a means of limiting the spread of contagious diseases, and introduced the method of risk factor analysis and the idea of a syndrome in the diagnosis of specific diseases.

(vi) Mesopotamian Concepts of Disease and Healing

Mesopotamian diseases are often blamed on pre-existing spirits: gods, ghosts, etc. However, each spirit was held responsible for only one of what we would call a disease in any one part of the body. So usually "Hand of God X" of the stomach corresponds to what we call a disease of the stomach. A number of diseases simply were identified by names, "bennu" for example. Also, it was recognised that various organs could simply malfunction, causing illness. Gods could also be blamed at a higher level for causing named diseases or malfunctioning of organs, although in some cases this was a way of saying that symptom X was not independent as usual, but was caused in this case by disease Y. It can also be shown that the plants used in treatment were generally used to treat the symptoms of the disease, and were not the sorts of things generally given for magical purposes to such a spirit. Presumably specific offerings were made to a particular god or ghost when it was considered to be a causative factor, but these offerings are not indicated in the medical texts, and must have been found in other texts.

Each of the above mentioned system has its philosophy of disease, health, body compositions and so on. In fact all these systems of medicine have philosophies and remedies regarding for birth control. The question of how effective and safe they are is a matter of research. Let us look into concepts of contraceptives–ancient perspectives.

CONCEPT OF CONTRACEPTIVES—ANCIENT PERSPECTIVE

Probably the oldest methods of contraception (aside from sexual abstinence) are *coitus interruptus*, certain barrier methods, and herbal methods (emmenagogues and abortifacients). *Coitus interruptus* (withdrawal of the penis from the vagina prior to ejaculation) probably predates any other form of birth control. Once the relationship between the emission of semen into the vagina and pregnancy was known or suspected, some men began to use this technique. This is not a particularly reliable method of contraception, as few men have the self-control to correctly practice the method at every single act of sexual intercourse. Although it is commonly believed that pre-ejaculate fluid can cause pregnancy, modern research has shown that pre-ejaculate fluid does not contain viable sperm.

There are historic records of Egyptian women using a pessary (a vaginal suppository) made of various acidic substances (crocodile dung is alleged) and lubricated with honey or oil, which may have been somewhat effective at killing sperm. However, it is important to note that the sperm cell was not discovered until Anton van Leeuwenhoek invented the microscope in the late 17th century, so barrier methods employed prior to that time could not know of the details of conception. Asian women may have used oiled paper as a cervical cap, and Europeans may have used beeswax for this purpose. The condom appeared sometime in the 17th century, initially made of a length of animal intestine. It was not particularly popular, nor as effective as modern latex condoms, but was employed both as a means of contraception and in the hopes of avoiding syphilis, which was greatly feared and devastating prior to the discovery of antibiotic drugs.

Various abortifacients have been used throughout human history, although many do not associate induced abortion with the term "birth control". Some of them were effective, some were not; those that were most effective also had major side effects. One abortifacient reported to have low levels of side effects — silphium — was harvested to extinction around the 1st century. The ingestion of certain poisons by the female can disrupt the reproductive system; women have drunk solutions containing mercury, arsenic, or other toxic substances for this purpose. The Greek gynaecologist Soranus in the 2nd century suggested that women drink water that blacksmiths had used to cool metal. The herbs tansy and pennyroyal are well-known in folklore as abortive agents, but these also "work" by poisoning the woman. Levels of the active chemicals in these herbs that will induce a miscarriage are high enough to damage the liver, kidneys, and other organs, making them very dangerous. However, in those times where risk of maternal death from postpartum complications was high, the risks and side effects of toxic medicines may have seemed less onerous. Some herbalists claim that black cohosh tea will also be effective in certain cases as an abortifacient.

The fact that various effective methods of birth control were known in the ancient world sharply contrasts with a seeming ignorance of these methods in wide segments of the population of early modern Christian Europe. This ignorance continued far into the 20th century, and was paralleled by eminently high birth rates in European countries during the 18th and 19th centuries. Some historians have attributed this to a series of coercive measures enacted by the emerging modern state, in an effort to repopulate Europe after the population catastrophe of the Black Death, starting in 1348. According to this view, the witch hunts were the first measure the modern state took in an attempt to eliminate knowledge about birth control within the population, and monopolise it in the hands of state-employed male medical specialists (gynaecologists). Prior to the witch hunts, male specialists were unheard of, because birth control was naturally a female domain.

Presenters at a family planning conference told a tale of Arab traders inserting small stones into the uteruses of their camels in order to prevent pregnancy, a concept very similar to the modern IUD. Although the story has been repeated as truth, it has no basis in history and was meant only for entertainment purposes.

Given this background let us new understand the concept of contraceptive from the modern or allopathic perspective.

CONCEPT OF CONTRACEPTIVES—MODERN PERSPECTIVE

Birth control is a regimen of one or more actions, devices, or medications followed in order to deliberately prevent or reduce the likelihood of a woman becoming pregnant or giving birth. For many people, birth control is an integral component of family planning. Mechanisms which are intended to reduce the likelihood of the fertilisation of an ovum by a spermatozoon may more specifically be referred to as *contraception*.

The first interuterine devices (which occupied both the vagina and the uterus) were first marketed around 1900. The first modern intrauterine device (contained entirely in the uterus) was described in a German publication in 1909, although the author appears to have never marketed his product.

The Rhythm Method (with a rather high method failure rate of ten per cent per year) was developed in the early 20th century, as researchers discovered that a woman only ovulates once per menstrual cycle. Not until the 1950s, when scientists better understood the functioning of the menstrual cycle and the hormones that controlled it, were methods of hormonal contraception and modern methods of fertility awareness (also called natural family planning) developed.

Barrier methods place a physical impediment to the movement of sperm into the female reproductive tract. The most popular barrier method is the male condom, a latex or polyurethane sheath placed over the penis. The condom is also available in a female version, which is made of polyurethane. The female condom has a flexible ring at each end — one secures behind the pubic bone to hold the condom in place, while the other ring stays outside the vagina.

Cervical barriers are devices that are contained completely within the vagina. The contraceptive sponge has a depression to hold it in place over the cervix. The cervical cap is the smallest cervical barrier. It stays in place by suction to the cervix or to the vaginal walls. The Lea's shield is a larger cervical barrier, also held in place by suction. The diaphragm fits into place behind the woman's pubic bone and has a firm but flexible ring, which helps it press against the vaginal walls.

The SILCS diaphragm is a new diaphragm design which is still in clinical testing and is not yet available.

Hormonal Methods

There is variety of delivery methods for hormonal contraception. Combinations of synthetic estrogens and progestin (synthetic progestogens) are commonly used. These include the combined oral contraceptive pill ("The Pill"), the Patch, and the contraceptive vaginal ring ("NuvaRing"). Not currently available for sale in the United States is Lunelle, a monthly injection.

Other methods contain only a progestin (a synthetic progestogen). These include the progestin only pill (the POP or 'minipill'), the injectables Depo Provera (a depot formulation of medroxyprogesterone acetate given as an intramuscular injection every three months) and Noristerat (norethisterone acetate given as an intramuscular injection every 8 weeks), and contraceptive implants. The progestin-only pill must be taken at more precisely remembered times each day than combined pills. The first contraceptive implant, the original 6-capsule Norplant, was removed from the market in the United States in 1999, though a newer single-rod implant called Implanon was approved for sale in the United States on July 17, 2006. The various progestin-only methods may cause irregular bleeding during use.

Ormeloxifene (Centchroman) is a selective oestrogen receptor modulator, or SERM. It causes ovulation to occur asynchronously with the formation of the uterine lining, preventing implantation of a zygote. It has been widely available as a birth control method in India since the early 1990s, marketed under the trade name Saheli. Centchroman is legally available only in India.

Intrauterine Methods

An intrauterine device: These are contraceptive devices which are placed inside the uterus. They are usually shaped like a "T" — the arms of the T hold the device in place. There are two main types of intrauterine contraceptives: those that contain copper (which has a spermicidal effect), and those that release a progestogen (in US the term progestin used).

The terminology used for these devices differs in the United Kingdom and the United States. In the US, all devices which are placed in the uterus to prevent pregnancy are referred to as Intra-Uterine Devices (IUDs). In the UK, only copper-containing devices are called IUDs, and hormonal intrauterine contraceptives are referred to with the term Intra-Uterine System (IUS). This may be because there are seven types of copper IUDs available in the UK, compared to only one in the US.

Emergency Contraception

Some combined pills and POPs may be taken in high doses to prevent pregnancy after a birth control failure (such as a condom breaking) or after unprotected sex. Hormonal emergency contraception is also known as the "morning after pill," although it is licensed for use up to three days after intercourse.

Copper intrauterine devices may also be used as emergency contraception. For this use, they must be inserted within five days of the birth control failure or unprotected intercourse. Because emergency contraception may prevent a fertilised egg from developing, some people consider it a form of abortion.

Induced abortion: Abortion can be done with surgical methods, usually suction-aspiration abortion (in the first trimester) or dilation and evacuation (in the second trimester).

Medical abortion uses drugs to end a pregnancy and is approved for pregnancies where the length of gestation has not exceeded 8 weeks.

Some herbs are believed to cause abortion (abortifacients). Peer-reviewed research has proven the efficacy of some of these substances, but the use of herbs to induce abortion is not recommended, due to the risk of serious side effects.

Sterilisation

Surgical sterilisation is available in the form of tubal ligation for women and vasectomy for men. In women, the process may be referred to as "tying the tubes," but the fallopian tubes may be tied, cut, clamped, or blocked. This serves to prevent sperm from joining the unfertilised egg. The non-surgical sterilisation procedure, is an example of a procedure that blocks the tubes. Sterilisation should be considered permanent.

Fertility Awareness Methods

Fertility Awareness (FA) methods involve a woman's observation and charting of one or more of her body's primary fertility signs, to determine the fertile and infertile phases of her cycle. Charting may be done by the woman on paper, with the assistance of software, or by fertility monitoring devices that accept and interpret temperature readings, information from home urinalysis tests, or both.

Unprotected sex is restricted to the least fertile period. During the most fertile period, barrier methods may be availed, or she may abstain from intercourse. Most methods track one or more of the three primary fertility signs: changes in basal body temperature, in cervical mucus, and in cervical position, though cervical position is most frequently used as a cross-reference with one or both of the others. If a woman tracks both basal body temperature and another primary sign, the method is referred to as *symptothermal*. Some fertility monitoring devices use urinalysis to follow the levels of estrogen and luteinising hormone throughout a woman's menstrual cycle. Other bodily cues such as mittelschmerz are considered secondary indicators.

The term *Natural Family Planning* (NFP) is sometimes used to refer to any use of FA methods. However, this term specifically refers to the practices which are permitted by the Roman Catholic Church — breastfeeding infertility, and periodic abstinence during fertile times. FA methods may be used by NFP users to identify these fertile times.

Statistical Methods

Statistical methods such as the Rhythm Method and Standard Days Method are dissimilar from observational fertility awareness methods, in that they do not involve the observation or recording of bodily cues of fertility. Instead, statistical methods estimate the likelihood of fertility based on the length of past menstrual cycles. Statistical methods are much less accurate than fertility awareness methods, and are considered by many fertility awareness teachers to have been obsolete for at least 20 years.

Coitus Interruptus

Coitus interruptus (literally "interrupted sex"), also known as the withdrawal method, is the practice of ending sexual intercourse ("pulling out") before ejaculation. The main risk of coitus interruptus is that the man may not make the maneuver in time. Although concern has been raised about the risk of pregnancy from sperm in pre-ejaculate, several small studies have failed to find any viable sperm in the fluid.

Avoiding Vaginal Intercourse

The risk of pregnancy from non-vaginal sex, such as outercourse (sex without penetration), anal sex, or oral sex is virtually zero. (A very small risk comes from the possibility of semen leaking onto the vulva (with anal sex) or coming into contact with an object, such as a hand, that later contacts the vulva.) However, with this method, care must be taken to prevent the progression to intercourse.

Abstinence

Sexual abstinence is the practice of refraining from all sexual activity.

Lactational

Most breastfeeding women have a period of infertility after the birth of their child. The lactational amenorrhea method, or LAM, gives guidelines for determining the length of a woman's period of breastfeeding infertility.

Methods in Development

For Females

Praneem is a polyherbal vaginal tablet being studied as a spermicide, and a microbicide active against HIV. Buffer-Gel is a spermicidal gel being studied as a microbicide active against HIV.

Duet is a disposable diaphragm in development that will be pre-filled with Buffer-Gel. It is designed to deliver microbicide to both the cervix and vagina. Unlike currently available diaphragms, the Duet will be manufactured in only one size and will not require a prescription, fitting, or a visit to a doctor.

The SILCS diaphragm is a silicone barrier which is still in clinical testing. It has a finger cup molded on one end for easy removal. Like the Duet, the SILCS is novel in that it will only be available in one size.

A vaginal ring is being developed that releases both estrogen and progesterone, and is effective for over 12 months.

Two types of progesterone-only vaginal rings are being developed. Progestogen-only products may be particularly useful for women who are breastfeeding. The rings may be used for four months at a time. Progesterone-only contraceptive is being developed that would be sprayed onto the skin once a day. Quinacrine sterilisation and the Adiana procedure are two permanent methods of birth control being developed.

For Males

Other than condoms and withdrawal, there are currently no available methods of reversible contraception which males can use or control. Several methods are in research and development:

As of 2007, a chemical called Adjudin is currently in Phase II human trials as a male oral contraceptive.

RISUG (Reversible Inhibition of Sperm Under Guidance), is an experimental injection into the vas deferens that coats the walls of the vas with a spermicidal substance. The method can potentially be reversed by washing out the vas deferens with a second injection.

Experiments in vas-occlusive contraception involve an implant placed in the vasa deferentia. Experiments in heat-based contraception involve heating a man's testicles to a high temperature for a short period of time.

Misconceptions

Modern misconceptions and urban legends have given rise to a great deal of false claims:

The suggestion that douching immediately following intercourse works as a contraceptive is untrue. While it may seem like a sensible idea to try to wash the ejaculate out of the vagina, it is not likely to be effective. Due to the nature of the fluids and the structure of the female reproductive tract – if anything, douching spreads semen further towards the uterus. Some slight spermicidal effect may occur if the douche solution is particularly acidic, but overall it is not scientifically observed to be a reliably effective method.

It is a myth that a female cannot become pregnant as a result of the first time she engages in sexual intercourse. While women are usually less fertile for the first few days of menstruation, it is a myth that a woman absolutely cannot get pregnant if she has sex during her period. Having sex in a hot tub does not prevent pregnancy, but may contribute to vaginal infections.

Although some sex positions may encourage pregnancy, no sexual positions prevent pregnancy. Having sex while standing up or with a woman on top will not keep the sperm from entering the uterus. The force of ejaculation, the contractions of the uterus caused by prostaglandins in the semen, as well as ability of sperm to swim overrides gravity.

Effectiveness is measured by how many women become pregnant using a particular birth control method in the first year of use. Thus, if 100 women use a method that has a 12 per cent first-year failure rate, then sometime during the first year of use, 12 of the women should become pregnant.

The most effective methods in typical use are those that do not depend upon regular user action. Surgical sterilisation, Depo-Provera, implants, and intrauterine devices (IUDs) all have first-year failure rates of less than one per cent for perfect use and typical use.

Other methods may be highly effective if used consistently and correctly, but can have typical use first-year failure rates that are considerably higher due to incorrect or ineffective usage by the user. Hormonal contraceptive pills, patches or rings, fertility awareness methods, and the lactational amenorrhoea method (LAM), if used strictly, have first-year (or for LAM, first-6-month) failure rates of less than 1 per cent. In one survey, typical use first-year failure rates of hormonal contraceptive pills (and by extrapolation, patches or rings) were as high as five per cent per year. Fertility awareness methods as a whole have typical use first-year failure rates as high as 25 per cent per year; however, as stated above, perfect use of these methods reduces the first-year failure rate to less than 1 per cent.

Condoms and cervical barriers such as the diaphragm have similar typical use first-year failure rates (14 and 20 per cent, respectively), but perfect usage of the condom is more effective (three per cent first-year failure versus six per cent) and condoms have the additional feature of helping to prevent the spread of sexually transmitted diseases such as the HIV virus. The withdrawal method, if used consistently and correctly, has a first-year failure rate of four per cent. Due to the difficulty of consistently using withdrawal correctly, it has a typical use first-year failure rate of 19 per cent and is not recommended by some medical professionals, although others believe it deserves more support.

TRADITIONAL AND MODERN PRACTICES— COMPARATIVE PERSPECTIVE

Contraception has been known to humankind from the earliest times. Ancient Jewish sources, early Islamic medical texts, and Hindu sacred scriptures all indicate that herbal contraceptives could induce temporary sterility. Today, however, there exists no uniform position on contraception within each of the major religious traditions; rather, the issue is marked by a plurality of views from followers, religious leaders and scholars. All of the traditions discussed below are founded on notions of fertility and procreation within the family and thus, while the views on contraception vary widely, no religion advocates the goal of a childless marriage or the use of contraception outside of the marriage contract.

Throughout history, mankind has tried to limit family size. Until the last century, this was largely achieved by behavioural modifications, including abstinence, infrequent coitus, the avoidance of intercourse during the fertile period of the cycle and coitus interruptus (the withdrawal method). In population terms, breast-feeding, which inhibits normal ovarian activity, has been one of the most important means of limiting fertility, whereas for individual couples, coitus interruptus – first mentioned in the book of Genesis – has had a major role to play. One artificial method of contraception, the condom, has a surprisingly long history. Penile sheaths were described in Egypt in 1350 BC. Originally made from animal intestines, and later from linen or silk, they were used mainly for protection from venereal disease. Not surprisingly, given the place of women in society, female barrier methods arrived much later on the contraceptive scene. The first 'womb veil' is attributed to an American working in the early 1800s and the first cervical cap was produced in Germany around 1830. It took more than 150 years before the female condom came on to the market in 1993.

Historically, many groups and societies have discouraged ***contraception*** (the prevention of conception, or birth control) to assure survival of its members and humanity as a whole. Certain religious groups strongly disapprove of sexual activity that does not culminate in coitus and the possibility of conception.

Other groups place little importance on the matter of contraception. The Yanomamo of South America, for instance, harbour little or no concept of contraception. Instead, they parent as many children as possible, and then kill off those they view as the undesirable, such as some females and deformed infants.

Modern medicine has spread throughout different parts of the world, and people of all ages now live longer, causing the world's population to explode in growth. In fact, at five billion today, the world's population doubles, on average, every 35 years, with most of this growth occurring in developing countries. Given this population crisis, certain governments, like that of China, regulate the number of births allowed per household.

Modern contraceptive methods have a surprisingly short history and are dominated by the oral contraceptive pill, which came on to the market in 1960. New developments since the advent of the pill have been largely limited to tinkering with the contents and routes of administration of hormonal contraception. The knowledge that would allow a more exciting approach to new contraceptives does exist but the will to proceed is hampered by financial, political and moral factors, and perhaps ironically by the AIDS epidemic.

The intrauterine device: Until the second half of the 20th century, the only other artificial method of contraception was the intrauterine device (IUD). It was first developed in 1909 in Germany from loops of silk–worm gut, later from silver–copper alloys and eventually from plastic. The modern IUD appeared in 1969 when copper was added to the plastic frame, improving contraceptive efficacy and allowing the size of the device to be reduced. Most recently, the plastic frame was removed in the belief that side-effects will be reduced through use of an even smaller device. IUDs fell into disrepute in the mid-70s when a rather fearsomely shaped device with a multifilament tail – the Dalkon Shield – was shown to be associated with pelvic infection and infertility. Nevertheless the IUD is one of the most commonly used methods of contraception in the world, thanks mainly to widespread use in China. Despite being highly effective, extremely safe, long-acting (IUDs are licensed for 5-10 years of use) and very cheap, the copper IUD is not popular in the USA, nor in much of Western Europe.

Advent of the oral contraceptive pill: The advent of the oral contraceptive pill, developed by Pincus and Rock and colleagues and first marketed in 1960, heralded a revolution in contraception and arguably laid the foundations for women's liberation. Perhaps the most widely researched drug in the history of therapeutics, the pill has been repeatedly shown to be safe and effective. It has been, and remains, a favourite subject of media hype, and despite its safety record, the majority of women still perceive the pill as potentially dangerous. It is of course statistically much safer than pregnancy.

Developments in oral contraception: Much of the very recent history of contraception centres round hormonal methods. In the first two decades after the pill was marketed, research efforts were concentrated on improving safety and reducing side effects. This was achieved by lowering the dose of estrogen (ethinylestradiol) and experimenting with different types of progesterone. The dose of estrogen has been reduced from 150_g to 20_g, and a pill containing 15_g is currently in clinical trials. Nervous of compromising efficacy with such a low dose, investigators have tried reducing the duration of the pill-free interval from the traditional seven days to four or five days and substituting the placebo tablet or pill-free day with a small dose of estrogen alone.

New routes of administration: Although the pharmaceutical industry still seems pre-occupied with the dose and type of steroids, research into hormonal contraception in the last twenty years has concentrated on the development of new delivery systems. Avoiding the oral route has the theoretical benefit of bypassing the first pass of metabolism through the liver and providing constant release rates of steroids. It has the very real benefits of reducing or eliminating the need for compliance and increasing choice. Progesterone-only contraceptive implants became widely available in the 1990s. Initially marketed as six silicon-rubber-coated rods that were implanted subdermally in the upper arm (Norplant), the number of rods was reduced to two (Norplant 2, Jadelle) and finally to one (Implanon). Implanon lasts for three years and to date no method failures have been reported. The addition of progesterone to the intrauterine device has produced an IUD that is licensed for 5 years, but which, in contrast to the copper IUD, is associated with a significant reduction in menstrual bleeding.

At the end of this long list of new delivery systems comes the contraceptive vaginal ring (worn in the vagina for 21 days and removed for 7 days) and a contraceptive trans-dermal patch. Both contain ethinylestradiol in combination with a progestogen and both will become available in the USA during 2002. Lagging behind (estrogen replacement therapy for menopausal women is already available in both forms) is the development of a trans-dermal gel and trans-nasal spray delivering contraceptive hormones. If and when these become available, all the different routes of administration of hormonal contraception will finally have been exhausted and perhaps technology will move on to something that is radically different.

Health Benefits of Contraception

The idea that contraception can be used not only to prevent pregnancy but also to confer health benefits, and particularly to reduce the frequency of menstrual bleeding, has received considerable interest in the last couple of years. However, this hypothesis is not new. It was demonstrated in the early 1970s in Scotland that women could, and would like to, run packets of oral contraceptive pills together, allowing a three-monthly, rather than a monthly, withdrawal bleed. The idea has recently been rediscovered in the USA, wherein 2002, a three-monthly combined oral contraceptive pill (Seasonale, Barr Laboratories, NJ) is in clinical trials.

The potential for additional health benefits may restore the enthusiasm of pharmaceutical companies for contraceptive research. The use of selective estrogen receptor modulators (SERMS), for example, to develop a contraceptive pill that reduces the risk of breast cancer must be very tempting.

Future Prospects

Although contraceptive development seems to have almost ground to a halt with regard to steroid hormone methods for women, some exciting work has been undertaken on some different technologies. The feasibility of hormonal contraception for men has been recognised for more than fifty years. It is, after all, based on the same concept as the pill. A variety of regimens have been tested, most of them (and probably the first to reach the market) comprising a progestogen to suppress spermatogenesis, combined with testosterone replacement to maintain sexual function. The long delay in the development of a hormonal method for men is due partly to the lack of an appropriate long-acting form of testosterone replacement, but also to the commonly held belief that 'men would never use it' and women would never trust them to take it. Although contraception is still very much seen as the responsibility of the woman, particularly in developing countries, recent surveys of men and women in Scotland, China, Hong Kong and South Africa suggest that a male pill would have a significant place in contraceptive choice. Lured by the potentially huge market of testosterone replacement therapy for ageing men, the pharmaceutical industry has at last made some, albeit not absolutely wholehearted, commitment to the development of hormonal contraception for men.

Immuno-contraception also seems to have been in the pipeline for a disproportionate length of time. Vaccination against the egg (specifically the zona pellucida), sperm and embryo (specifically, human chorionic gonadotropin) are all technically possible. However, progress has been hampered by a variety of factors, including uncertainty about the long-term effects of immunising against human tissues, and fears, perhaps ironically from women's groups that contraceptive vaccines too easily lend themselves to coercive family planning policies.

Perhaps the greatest promise for a radically new method lies with the use of anti-progesterone. Orally active and effective as a daily or once-a-month pill, the anti-progesterone mifepristone is now marketed in China as an emergency contraceptive. Elsewhere in the world, its development has been seriously inhibited by the anti-abortion lobby, because the principal use of mifepristone is as an abortion pill. The saga of mifepristone illustrates the difficulties that almost every advance in contraception has encountered. It may seem obvious, but contraception cannot be separated from sex, and everyone is interested in sex. Thus, in contrast to, say, anti-hypertensive drugs, everyone tends to have a view on contraception. Contraception is also inextricably bound up with social, cultural, moral and religious factors that often influence, if not the availability of methods, certainly their accessibility. The increasing tendency towards litigation, which even if unsuccessful, is extraordinarily expensive and time-consuming, has also served as a damper on the development and availability of new methods. All these influences make the pharmaceutical industry nervous when it comes to taking on new leads.

Impediments to Contraceptive Development

In recent years, research progress has depended largely on not-for-profit organisations, such as the World Health Organisation and the Population Council. However, two significant factors have had a major effect on even their enthusiasm to develop new methods. The first is the HIV/AIDS epidemic. Although it led to the renaissance of the condom and a renewed interest in the development of better barrier methods, albeit with limited scope for much improvement, it has undoubtedly reduced the interest in developing other new methods of contraception. This is partly because funds and research efforts have been sidetracked into developing microbicides, but also because of the commonly-held view that it is bordering on the 'unethical' to work on new methods of contraception that do not simultaneously prevent HIV transmission.

The second major impediment to contraceptive development has been the widespread view that the population problem has been solved, with the result that donors no longer regard contraceptive research as a priority. It is indeed true that in the thirty years between 1965 and 1995 the total fertility rate (TFR) in the world fell from 4.9 to 2.8 children per woman and that in 1997, 51 countries – accounting for over 44 per cent of the global population – had fertility rates below the replacement level. However, the TFR in most countries of the African continent is over 5.5, and in these same countries less than 20 per cent of married women are using contraception. Despite higher contraceptive prevalence, abortion rates continue to rise in most countries worldwide, including the developed world, and unwanted and mis-timed pregnancy accounts for tens of thousands of maternal deaths each year.

GLOBAL POLICIES OF THE WORLD HEALTH ORGANISATION

The main objectives of the WHO traditional medicine activities are:

- To facilitate integration of traditional medicine into the national health care system by assisting Member States to develop their own national policies on traditional medicine;
- To promote the proper use of traditional medicine by developing and providing international standards, technical guidelines and methodologies;
- To act as a clearing-house to facilitate information exchange in the field of traditional medicine.

The objective of the strategy is to discuss the role of traditional medicine in health care systems, current challenges and opportunities and WHO's role and strategy for traditional medicine. Many Member States and many of WHO's partners in traditional medicine (UN agencies, international organisations, non-governmental organisations, and global and national professional associations) contributed to the Strategy and have expressed their willingness to participate in its implementation. The Strategy was reviewed by the WHO Cabinet in July 2001 and, based on Cabinet comments, has since been revised. The Strategy was printed in January 2002. Since this is at present a working document, the proposed objectives and activities have started to be implemented in early 2002 and the Strategy will be widely disseminated. We understand that the situation in the use of traditional medicine is quite different from country to country and region to region. For example, in AFRO and in WPRO, the Member States consider that traditional medicine is a priority for health care in their regions, but in other regions the role of traditional medicine is treated as complementary or alternative medicine.

Use of plant based drugs and chemicals for curing various ailments and personal adornment is as old as human civilisation. In India, the sacred Vedas dating back between 3500 B.C and 800 B.C give many references of medicinal plants. One of the remotest works in traditional herbal medicine is "*Virikshayurveda*", compiled even before the beginning of Christian era and formed the basis of medicinal studies in ancient India. "Rig Veda", one of the oldest Indian literatures written around 2000 B.C. mentions the use of Cinnamon (Cinnamomum verum Prel.), Ginger (Zingiber officinale Rose.), Sandalwood (Santalum album L.) etc. not only in religious ceremonies but also in medical preparation (Bentley and Trimen, 1980). Plants and plant-based medicaments are the basis of many of the modern pharmaceuticals we used today for our various ailments (Abraham, 1981; Atal and Kapur, 1982). At one time, nearly all medicines were derived from biological resources. Even today they remain vital and as much as 67 per cent-70 per cent of modern medicines are derived from natural products (State of the Environment Report, 2001). Nearly 80 per cent of the world populations rely on traditional medicines for primary health care, most of which involve the use of plant extracts (Sandhya et al., 2006). In India, almost 95 per cent of the prescriptions are plant-based in the traditional systems of Unani, Ayurveda, Homoeopathy and Siddha (Satyavati et al., 1987).

Ancient ethnic communities around the world had learnt to utilise their neighbourhood herbal flora for various curative as well as offensive purposes (Subramoniam and Pushpangadan, 1995). Due to lack of literacy, their knowledge on plants developed often at the cost of their dear life through centuries old experience could not be perfectly documented and it had rather descended from one generation to another as a domestic cultural heritage. As the ethnic groups migrated from place to place in search of their livelihood, their folklore knowledge also became fragmented and travelled with them often with 'additions and deletions'. Their findings in course of time have become basic leads for chemical, pharmacological, clinical and biochemical investigations, which ultimately gave birth to drug discovery.

When one is in charge of defining the concept of traditional medicine, one realises the complexity of such a task, as situations actually vary accordingly to countries and populations taken into consideration. Traditional medicine constitutes an extremely fascinating and attractive world under many points of view, and for a wide range of users in developing and developed countries. For example, traditional medicine may be either highly secretive, mystical and extremely localised, or codified and very well regulated. As a consequence, traditional medical knowledge may be passed on orally from generation to generation or may be openly taught in officially recognised universities.

However, the WHO has delineated a working definition of traditional medicine as "including diverse health practices, approaches, knowledge and beliefs incorporating plant, animal, and/or mineral based medicines, spiritual therapies, manual techniques and exercises applied singularly or in combination to maintain well-being, as well as to treat, diagnose or prevent illness".

Furthermore, traditional medicine therapies can be categorised as medication therapies, when they use herbal medicines, animal parts and/or minerals, and as non-medication therapies, if carried out mainly without the use of medication, as in the case of acupuncture or manual therapies.

The term traditional medicine is sometimes replaced by other terms, as complementary, alternative or non-conventional medicine. The different terminology is frequently used in countries where traditional medicine is practiced even though it is not part of the country's own tradition, or if it is not integrated into its dominant health care system. If allopathic medicine refers to the broad category of medical practice that is sometimes called Western medicine, biomedicine, scientific medicine or modern medicine, the adjective complementary, alternative and non-conventional refer to health care that is considered supplementary to allopathic medicine.

This categorisation depends on the health care system of the country taken into consideration. The WHO individuates basically three types of health system with the aim of describing the degree to which traditional medicine is an officially recognised element of health care:

Integrative system: Traditional medicine is officially recognised and incorporated into all areas of health care provision (health care delivery, education, training, regulation, insurance). This happens for example in China, Republic of Korea and Vietnam.

Inclusive system: Traditional medicine is recognised, but it is not yet completely integrated into all aspects of health care. This system is typical of countries such as United Kingdom, USA, Canada, Norway, Germany, Australia, and also Nigeria, India, Ghana, Indonesia, Sri Lanka, Japan and United Arab Emirates.

Tolerant system: The national health care system is totally based on allopathic medicine. However some traditional medicine practices are tolerated by law. This is, for example, the case of Italy.

The most widespread systems of traditional medicine in the world are Chinese medicine.

The earliest record of traditional medicine can be trace back to the 8th century B.C.. Diagnosis and treatment are based on a holistic view of the patient's symptoms, expressed in terms of the balance of yin and yang. Yin represents the earth, cold and femininity. Yang represents the sky, heat and masculinity. The actions of yin and yang influence the interactions of the five elements composing the universe: metal, wood, water, fire and earth. Practitioners of Chinese medicine seek to control the levels of yin and yang through 12 meridians, which bring energy to the body. Acupuncture, for example, that is one of the most widely used Chinese medicine practices, is based on the meridian theory. Herbal medicines are also a consistent part of such a traditional system.

Ayurveda's origin can be dated back even earlier, in the 10th century B.C. However, its current form took shape between the 5th century B.C. and the 5th century A.D. The term ayurveda is a Sanskrit term meaning 'science of life', and in fact, ayurveda is not only a system of medicine, but also a way of living. Ayurvedic philosophy is linked to sacred texts, the Vedas, and based on the theory of *Panchamahabhutas*. All objects and living bodies are composed of the five basic elements: earth, water, fire, air and sky. Furthermore, the environment is perceived as a macrocosm, and the individual as a microcosm, reciprocally acting on each other.

Ayurveda is widely practiced in South Asia, especially in Bangladesh, India, Nepal, Pakistan, and Sri Lanka.

Chiropractic: Chiropractic was more recently founded at the end of the 19th century. The founder was a magnetic therapist practicing in Iowa, USA, named Daniel David Palmer. This therapy is based on an association between the spine and nervous system and on the self-healing properties of the human body. It diagnoses and treats mechanical disorders of the joints, muscles and ligaments of the body by manual adjustments.

Homoeopathy: Homoeopathy was first mentioned by Hippocrates (462-377 B.C.), but it was a German physician, Hahnemann (1755-1843), who established homoeopathy's basic principles, among which the most important is 'simila similibus curentur'. The founder wrote that "in order to radically heal a certain kind of chronic infections, it is necessary to find remedies which normally cause in the human body a similar disease, as much similar as possible". Basically this means that a substance, which absorbed in a certain quantity in a healthy person may cause a disease, may also cure it if taken in a different dose. Other principles are direction of cure, principle of single remedy, the theory of minimum diluted dose, and the theory of chronic diseases.

Homoeopathy is widely diffuse in Europe, as well as in Asia and in North America. It has also been integrated in the systems of many countries, including India, Mexico, Pakistan, Sri Lanka, and the United Kingdom.

Unani: Unani is based on Hippocrates' theory of the four bodily humours: blood, phlegm, yellow bile, and black bile. Galen (131-210 A.D.), Rhazes (850-925 A.D.) and Avicenna (980-1037 A.D.) heavily influenced unani's foundation and formed its structure. Unani is therefore Greek medicine which developed throughout the Arabic civilisation. It draws from the traditional systems of medicine of China, Egypt, India, Iraq, Persia, and the Syrian Arabi Republic. It is also called Arabic medicine.

The use of traditional medicine in the prevention, diagnosis and treatment of an extensive range of diseases, has been increasing, overall in the last 20 years, both in developing and developed countries.

Source: WHO Traditional Medicine Strategy 2002-2005, p. 9

The reasons for such popularity are different accordingly to the countries taken into consideration.

In developing countries, traditional medicine is considered more accessible and affordable than allopathic medicine. To give an example, 80 per cent of the population in Africa uses traditional medicine. According to a survey by the US Agency for International Development, in Sub-Saharan Africa, traditional practitioners outnumber allopathic practitioners by 100 to 1. Furthermore, allopathic practitioners are usually located in cities or other urban areas. Traditional medicine, then, becomes for rural population the only source of health care.

Traditional medicine sometimes also constitutes the only affordable source of health care. This is why herbal medicines are mainly used to cure malaria (Artemisia annua), and are also used to obtain symptomatic relief and to manage opportunistic infections in patients affected by HIV/AIDS.

In developed countries, traditional medicine is perceived as a diverse approach to ill-health. Traditional medicine is based on "the needs of individuals. Different people may receive different treatments even if, according to modern medicine, they suffer from the same disease. Traditional medicine is based on a belief that each individual has his or her own constitution and social circumstances which result in different reactions to 'causes of disease' and 'treatment'". For this reason, the increasing use of traditional medicine arises from the dissatisfaction caused by the allopathic medicine approach.

Moreover, as we have previously seen, non-communicable diseases have been tremendously growing in developed countries. Even if allopathic medicine provides the patients with multiple treatments and technologies, this approach has not been sufficiently effective. For many patients, traditional medicine sometime offers gentler means to manage such diseases, to improve the quality of life of persons living with chronic diseases, as well as for the ageing population.

The Action taken by the WHO

The increasing diffusion of the use of traditional medicine in the world has been asking for the World Health Organisation's intervention. Member states' requests insistently reach WHO every day. Member states want assistance from WHO in formulating national policy and regulatory frameworks about traditional medicine; in ensuring the safety, efficacy and quality of the practices; in guaranteeing the access to such treatments and in assuring their rational use.

Dr. Samba, WHO's Regional Director for Africa, comments that if 80 per cent of the people in Africa really uses traditional medicine, "we must move quickly to evaluate its safety, efficacy, quality and standardisation — to protect our heritage and to preserve our traditional knowledge. We must also institutionalise and integrate it into our national health systems".

Problems have also arisen in the past from the improper use of traditional medicine. For example, in 1996, in Belgium, more than 50 people suffered kidney failure after taking herbal preparation which contained Aristolochia fangchi (a toxic plant) instead of Stephania tetranda or Magnolia officinalis.

Within the WHO, the structure entitled of responding to such challenges is the Traditional Medicine Team, in the Essential Drugs and Medicine Policies Department, Health and Pharmaceuticals Cluster. The basic objectives of the Traditional Medicine Team are: to facilitate integration of traditional medicine into the national health care system by assisting member states to develop their own national policies on traditional medicine; to promote the proper use of traditional medicine by developing and providing international standards, technical guidelines and methodologies; to study the potential usefulness of traditional medicine including evaluation of practices and examination of the safety and efficacy of remedies; to act as a clearing-house to facilitate information exchange in the field of traditional medicine; to educate and inform the general practices about proven traditional health practices.

One of the highest achievements of the Traditional Medicine Team's work has been the formulation of the first five-year strategy for traditional medicine, namely 'WHO Traditional Medicine Strategy 2002-2005 issued in May 2002. For the release of the document, the Traditional Medicine Team has received the contribution from numerous member states and partners, such as organisations of the UN system, international organisations, non-governmental organisations and global and national professional associations.

The Strategy has four main objectives:

Policy: to integrate relevant aspects of traditional medicine within national health care systems by framing national traditional medicine policies and implementing programmes;

Safety, efficacy and quality: to promote the safety, efficacy and quality of traditional medicine practices by providing guidance on regulatory and quality assurance standards;

Access: to increase access to, and affordability of, traditional medicine;

Rational use: to promote rational use of traditional medicine.

Source: WHO Traditional Medicine Strategy 2002-2005, p. 45.

Concerning the implementation of such objectives, the strategy proposes:

Policy

A policy is "a commitment to a goal and a guide to action". Even if only 25 of WHO's 192 member states (as of 2000) have developed national policies on traditional medicine, they are actually necessary tools in order to define the role of traditional medicine in the health care system, and its good employ. In general, such policy should cover a range of issues, such as: the definition of the government's role in developing traditional medicine in the health-care delivery system; provisions for safety and quality assurance; provisions for education and training; provisions for research and development; and also consideration of intellectual property issues.

A useful document in this sense, collecting data about legal frameworks worldwide, was issued in 2001 regarding to the 'Legal status of traditional medicine and complementary/ alternative medicine.

Safety, Efficacy, Quality

Differently from allopathic medicine that has developed mainly within the Western culture, traditional medicine has rather been influenced by different cultures and historical conditions. Furthermore, its common basis being a holistic approach to life, traditional medicine takes into accounts multiple and various factors. Its nature, therefore, renders it difficult to be evaluated, since there are no common standards and methods to do so.

WHO's task consists, then, in assuring safety, efficacy and quality of traditional medicine through increasing the knowledge about the various practices, and developing norms, standards and guidelines. An example is the regulation of herbal medicine, and the 'Guidelines on basic training and safety in acupuncture'. Another initiative should be the adoption of a national expert committee. For example, in the African Region, 21 out of 46 countries have institutes carrying out research in traditional medicine.

Access

To guarantee access to traditional medicine means to ensure its equitable availability and affordability, with a particular attention to the poorest population. In low-income countries, the need of inexpensive and effective treatments for common diseases is very high. Yet one-third, and sometimes even a half of the population of these countries, lack regular access to essential drugs. Traditional medicine is, in comparison, much more available and affordable than allopathic medicine.

With the purpose of increasing the access to traditional medicine, first, reliable indicators to accurately measure levels of access – both financial and geographic – to it must be developed; and, secondly, the safest and most effective therapies must be identified, to provide a sound basis for efforts to promote it.

It should also be considered that traditional practitioners live at the community level, making traditional medicine extremely available. For this reason, "the role of traditional practitioners should be recognised and cooperation between them and community health-workers should be strengthened".

Other issues are the protection of traditional knowledge, which has been increasingly appropriated, adapted and patented by scientists and industry, and sustainable use of natural resources, which sometimes are being wastefully exploited. A method which can be adopted to protect traditional medicine is to create national inventory of medicinal plants to ensure that knowledge is correctly and continuously used over generations. An example is the survey among traditional practitioners conducted by the Ministry of Health of Cote d'Ivoire that recorded more than 2000 traditionally use plants. The sustainable use of medical plants is, for example, improved by the project of the Traditional Medicine Team relatively to 'Good Sourcing Practice for Medicinal Plant'.

Rational Use

To guarantee rational use of medicines means generally to ensure sound and cost-effective use of drugs by health professionals and consumers. Regarding to traditional medicine, in particular, rational use has many aspects: proper use of good-quality products; good communication between traditional medicine providers; provision of scientific information and guidance for the public.

There are various challenges the WHO should face. With respect to education and training, the WHO should ensure that knowledge, qualification and training of traditional medicine providers are adequate. In addition, the WHO should also make traditional medicine and allopathic practitioners understand and appreciate the complementarities of the two different approaches.

Furthermore, the proper use of good quality products also contributes to guarantee rational use of traditional medicine.

Another element is to provide consumers with the necessary information in order to raise awareness of safe and appropriate use of traditional medicines. WHO's interventions should therefore be targeted both to providers and consumers. The WHO should work for increasing the capacity of traditional providers to use traditional medicine properly, and to increase the capacity of consumers to make informed decisions about traditional medicine.

Traditional Medicine and WHO's Mandate

Once analysed the fascinating world of traditional medicine and, in particular, the role of the Traditional Medicine Team within the WHO, this last section is aimed at understanding once more why the Organisation is engaged in such an activity. It is again a question on WHO's mandate.

First of all, what has traditional medicine to do with the development promoted by the Millennium Development Goals? Traditional medicine, as previously said, is on a wide range used by the poorest population of the world in developing countries. The reasons are its accessibility and affordability in comparison with allopathic medicine. Therefore, with no doubt, a correct use of such therapies and practices would be able to lead to the development of those people. Moreover, traditional medicine can properly be used in case of communicable diseases such as malaria and HIV, and in maternal health through traditional birth attendance. On this perspective, such a WHO activity responds to the fifth and sixth Millennium Development Goals. Secondly, traditional medicine seems to be perfectly in accordance with the definition of health given by the WHO Constitution, and it fits with the strategic objective of 'Health for All'.

Traditional medicine is based on "a holistic approach to life, equilibrium between the mind, body and their environment, and an emphasis on health rather than on disease". Such a unique vision, which is not at all common in the Western 'scientific' approach to health, is in the pathway designed by the constitutional definition of health, which goes beyond the mere absence of disease and introduces a state of complete physical, mental and social well-being.

Moreover, the use of traditional medicine as a response to primary health care needs, above all in the poorest population, makes it one of the most useful means to reach the Health for All objectives. The achievement of such an objective requires the employment of all the resources available in the world at any kind of level. Within this category, traditional medicine is absolutely a resource which should not be wasted and rather properly utilised.

Furthermore, one does not have to forget that traditional medicine also plays a role in developed countries were people are mostly affected by non-communicable diseases and, in particular, by chronic illnesses. For its holistic approach to health, it also highlights the importance of prevention, and of maintaining a certain style of life avoiding risk factors. Fròm this point of view, traditional medicine can contribute to improve the quality of life of those who suffer from minor illness or from certain incurable diseases. The reference, with this perspective, is to more than one of the strategic direction of the corporate strategy.

To summarise, traditional medicine can be employed on a variety of different fronts: it is actually used in developing and developed countries, and for treating both communicable and non-communicable diseases. This characteristic elevates traditional medicine to a universal level that makes it object of interest of an international organisation as WHO.

Nevertheless, the structure within the WHO, aimed at supporting the enormous possibility of employment of traditional medicine, shows a paradox. Despite the huge amount of work which could be done within this context in order to collect precious fruits, the Traditional Medicine Team is tied up by a ridiculous budget which does not even allow it to hire the needed personnel.

The budget of the Essential Medicines Department: access, quality and rational use is very little in comparison with that one of the previous analysed activities, and it does not seem to be dramatically increasing. Delaying reproduction is important in influencing population growth rates. Over a period of 60 years, if people delay reproduction until they are 30 years old, you would have only two generations, while if you do not delay reproduction you would have three generations (one generation every 20 years). The government's commitment to decreasing population growth creates policies that help decreasing the number of children being born.

The policies that contribute to the slowing of population growth are tested and cost-effective. Improving access to a range of high-quality contraceptive services remains a central strategy for closing the gap between reproductive intentions and outcomes. Lack of such access is a primary reason that today nearly two out of every five pregnancies are unintended, and that more than 150 million women do not want to become pregnant but are not using any form of contraception. Similarly, making sure that all girls and boys everywhere complete secondary school not only improves human development and health outcomes, but also discourages early and frequent pregnancy and thus contributes powerfully to slower population growth. The same is true of improving opportunities for women to find paying jobs or start their own businesses.

International agreements provide benchmarks for performance in these areas. In particular, governments should support and fund the social investments called for by the Programme of Action of the ICPD, which both focus on women's well-being and promise to contribute to slower population growth and the conservation of critical natural resources. When projecting future changes in environmental conditions, environmental and policy analysts should take into account scenarios suggested by the full range of population projections published by the United Nations Population Division and others, rather than merely those based on middle projections. Both governments and non-governmental organisations should consider integrated, global community-based approaches that improve both natural-resource conservation and access to reproductive health services.

Birth control in any method, technique, practice, device, or drug which is used to reduce the probability of pregnancy or to end an unwanted pregnancy. The term family planning is sometimes also used, especially when referring to the thoughtful and premeditated selection of a birth control technique.

When pregnancy is not desired, at least one of the participants must be sterile, sexual intercourse must be avoided, or *contraception* must be used prior to conception.

Contraception (even vasectomy) is not always 100 per cent effective. More generally, in sexual behaviour contact of semen with the vagina should be avoided. For example, partners can restrict themselves to masturbation, oral sex, etc., but they should not forget to keep not only the penis but also the sperm away from the vagina. Abstinence is sometimes called the only 'sure' way to avoid pregnancy. If perfectly adhered to, it is. However, some who habitually rely on it as their primary protection may cease to abstain and thereby incur the risk of pregnancy.

UNFPA promotes the human right of every woman, man and child to enjoy a life of health and equal opportunity. In many parts of the world, extreme poverty subjects women and men to a lack of real choices, opportunities and the basic services needed to improve their situations. Women often suffer disproportionately, due to violence, discrimination and the burden of poor reproductive health, which is the leading cause of death and disability for women in their reproductive years.

Every minute, one woman dies during pregnancy and birth because she did not receive adequate care and prompt treatment. By increasing interventions for safe motherhood, we can save the lives of half a million women and seven million infants, each year, and at the same time prevent millions of women from suffering from infections, injury and disability.

Perhaps nowhere is the need for reproductive health services more urgent than in the fight against HIV/AIDS. Every day, 6,800 people are newly infected, and about half are young people under the age of 25. Many know little about the disease and how the virus is transmitted. Young women are especially vulnerable and are more likely to be infected than young men. Reproductive health services that empower women and young people with life-saving information and skills will help prevent HIV from spreading and reduce further suffering and social and economic disruption.

UNFPA supports countries in using data for policies and programmes to address the complex linkages between population dynamics, poverty and sustainable development. Directing more resources to all of these issues is critical to meeting the Millennium Development Goals, the internationally agreed framework to halve poverty by the year 2015.

U.N. plans ways to limit births: the United Nations population fund supports abortion and sterilisation programmes throughout the third world and is seeking to impose birth-control methods as human rights - Nation: population control.

Maternal-and infant-mortality rates in the United States have decreased dramatically this century with the development of modern obstetrics and improvements in health care for women. Not so, however, in the developing world: Anaemia, malaria, obstructed labour when giving birth, haemorrhage, postpartum infection and lack of trained medical professionals are the major causes of maternal mortality. Meanwhile, according to the World Health Organisation, or WHO, 15 children die every minute as a result of disease and malnutrition.

The United Nations long has been concerned about these issues and has tied them to population control and economic development. At the end of June, a special session of the U.N. General Assembly will meet in New York to review implementation of the action programme of the 1994 Cairo Conference on Population and Development. The U.N. Population Fund (previously known as the U.N. Fund for Population Activities, or UNFPA) is the sponsoring U.N. secretariat. The conference document recommended global policies on world population, development, migration, gender equality, empowerment of women, access to family planning and reproductive health care.

Surprisingly, 179 countries signed off on the original action programme. Not surprisingly, five years later, not all are happy with the implementation.

POLICIES OF THE GOVERNMENT OF INDIA

A specific population policy for the tribal communities based on ethics of voluntarism with support for not only for the economic and health needs of the community members, but also for addressing critical issues like socio-cultural norms, land rights, migration and most importantly, gender power relations.

A Population Policy for Tribal Communities based on the Ethics of Voluntarism the development of a policy response to the pro-natalist behaviour has to be culturally sensitive and based on ethical approach. The ethical basis of the Indian population policy is that of voluntarism which should address not only the economic and health needs of the community members, but also critical issues like socio-cultural norms, migration and most importantly gender power relations. But India's population programmes have fallen far short in terms of integrating their objectives with the socio-cultural needs of the people, especially in tribal communities where members are increasingly feeling threatened by a perceived 'identity loss'.

The population programmes have been confronted with the dilemma of 'target oriented goals' and the maintaining of their 'ethical base', but at the end there should not be any compromise in addressing the programme objectives on an ethical basis. Without such a commitment, there will be a growing demographic disparity in India, which like economic disparities will end up as a matter of grave concern for planners and policy-makers.

This demographic disparity leading to demographic imbalance may cause considerable social turbulence and may even pose a threat to political stability. Demographers must look far beyond demographic statistics and anticipate the consequences of a demographic imbalance between different regions and states in India as well as between different religious communities, castes and tribes (Bose 1996). Although India has implemented various population programmes in the last fifty years, surprisingly it has not had a national population policy until as recently as the year 2000.

In spite of the fact that India was the first country in the world to officially begin a national family planning programme, it was largely an urban clinic-based programme rather than a policy with long-term objectives. During all the years prior to the release of a comprehensive national population policy, various statements of national-level population policy were advanced, but never adopted. When the National Health Policy was adopted in 1983, Parliament called for a separate policy on population, but it was never actually formulated. The backlash generated by the coercive programme of mass sterilisation during the mid-1970s created a fear among the politicians of being associated publicly with the subject of population for at least the next two decades. Statements of National Population Policy were made in 1976. In 1993 the Karunakaran Report (Report of the National Development Council (NDC) Committee on Population) proposed the formulation of a National Population Policy to take a long term holistic view of development, population growth and environmental protection (Government of India 2000, p.30). Accordingly the policy statements of 1976 were placed on the table.

However, the Parliament never really discussed or adopted them (Planning Commission 1992 in Government of India 2000, p.30). But before the 1994 Cairo International Conference on Population and Development (ICPD), the Government of India appointed an expert group under the chairmanship of the renowned scientist Dr. M.S. Swaminathan to develop a draft national population policy. The draft called for a radical shift to a policy that would be 'pro-poor, pro-woman, and pro-nature'. The draft also argued for a more bottom-up and needs-based approach that would be implemented by a new and powerful National Commission on Population (Sen 2000). The draft was again never formalised and no policy document was adopted. But after the ICPD the Government in 1996 formally abolished contraceptive targets. In 1997 (the 50th anniversary of India's Independence) the Cabinet approved the draft but again the document could not be tabled in either House of Parliament (Government of India 2000, p. 31). In the year 2000, National Population Policy was finally passed by the National Parliament.

Fortunately, the 'National Population Policy (NPP) 2000' seems to be attempting to move in a more humane direction (Sen 2000). The NPP 2000 has rightly emphasised a more ethical approach by downplaying to some extent the 'incentive/disincentive approach' that existed in earlier population programmes. Empowerment of women gets special mention in the action plan of the NPP 2000. The strategic themes of the National Population Policy emphasise the role of panchayats (local governing bodies at the village level) and zila parishads (local governing bodies at the district level) in promoting a gender sensitive, multi-sectoral agenda for population stabilisation, that will think, plan and act locally with support nationally. Moreover, the NPP also recognises the need for panchayats to be headed by women to identify area-specific unmet needs for reproductive health services, and prepare needs-based, demand-driven, socio-demographic plans at the village level aimed at identifying and providing responsive, people-centered and integrated, basic reproductive and child health care (Government of India 2000).

While these strategic themes in NPP 2000 can be welcomed without any hesitation, their implementation is highly questionable. The question of cultural identity or cultural survival is a growing concern for most of the tribal communities of our country. A population policy for tribal communities in India needs to address this issue with the utmost care and suitability.

Gaps in Policies

The Draft National Policy on Tribals of the Government of India states that the thrust of the Nehruvian policy is to respect the tribal peoples' rights in land and forest. However, in the implementation of the programmes for the indigenous and tribal peoples, there has been little application of the rights—the main reason for the failure, in the words of Draft National Policy on Tribals, to "translate the constitutional provisions into a reality". The rights based approaches i.e. incorporation of the rights accorded to the indigenous and tribal peoples under the constitution and various laws in the development of policies and implementation of programmes concerning them are indispensable if the Draft National Policy is to have any meaning.

Unfortunately, the programme of actions suggested in the Draft National Policy on Tribals do not incorporate rights-based approaches. The Government of India continues with charity approach. Many of the measures included in the National Policy including education in mother tongues of the indigenous and tribal children were raised in the first Five Year Plan for 1951-1956. Obviously the programmes have failed. There is simply no reference to the recommendations made in the evaluations and studies of the Programmes Evaluation Organisation of the Planning Commission of India and the Joint Parliamentary Committee on the Welfare of the Scheduled Castes and Scheduled Tribes about the existing policies, programmes and laws concerning the indigenous and tribal peoples.

The failure of the programmes to bring indigenous and tribal peoples at par with the general population and increasing marginalisation of indigenous and tribal peoples are reflected from increasing gap in education. According to the census figures, the gap between the general population including the Scheduled Castes and the Scheduled Tribes was 18.15 per cent in 1971, 19.88 per cent in 1981 and 22.61 per cent in 1991. Since the Scheduled Tribes, who constituted about 8.1 per cent of the total populations according to 1991 census, are also included in the general population, in actual terms, the gap in the literacy rate is much higher.

Although the female literacy rate of indigenous/tribal peoples has increased substantially from 4.85 per cent in 1971 to 18.9 per cent in 1991, the gap between indigenous females and the general female has been widening with 13.84 per cent in 1971, 21.81 per cent in 1981 and 21.10 per cent in 1991. The increase in literacy rate of the indigenous and tribal peoples, in particular female literacy rate, at all India level can be attributed to the high rate of literacy in North East India. The literacy rate of the indigenous and tribal populations in Madhya Pradesh according to 1991 census was 21.54 per cent with female literacy rate of 10.73 per cent. However, the literacy rate according to 1991 census was 41.59 per cent in Arunachal Pradesh, 52.89 per cent in Assam, 59.89 per cent in Manipur, 49.10 per cent in Meghalaya, 82.27 per cent in Mizoram, 61.65 per cent in Nagaland and 60.44 per cent in Tripura. The female literacy rate according to 1991 census was 29.69 per cent in Arunachal Pradesh, 43.03 per cent in Assam, 47.60 per cent in Manipur, 44.85 in Nagaland, 78.60 per cent in Mizoram, 54.75 in Nagaland and 49.65 per cent in Tripura.

The drop-out rate among indigenous and tribal peoples is very alarming. Various steps taken by the State governments to check drop out including free distribution of books and stationery, scholarship, reimbursement of examination fee, free bus travel etc have failed. The Joint Parliamentary Committee on the Welfare of Scheduled Castes and Scheduled Tribes of the 13th Lok Sabha in its 23rd Report of February 2003 on the working of Integrated Tribal Development Projects in Rajasthan reported that the delay in disbursement of scholarships is one of the reasons for increasing drop-out of indigenous and tribal students. No evaluation of the programmes on education including the Ashram schools under the Tribal Sub-Plan (TSP) was conducted so as to understand the shortcomings and suggest corrective measures.

The standards of health of indigenous and tribal peoples remain deplorable. The Joint Parliamentary Committee on the Welfare of Scheduled Castes and Scheduled Tribes of the 13th Lok Sabha in its 23rd Report of February 2003 stated that hundreds of posts of medical staff in Tribal Sub-Plan areas in Rajasthan have been lying vacant. The State government of Rajasthan could not give any answer as to the reasons for not filling up the vacancies.

In its Eighth Report of November 2000, the Joint Parliamentary Committee on the Welfare of Scheduled Castes and Scheduled Tribes of the 13th Lok Sabha stated that the actual requirement of doctors in tribal areas/scheduled areas in Madhya Pradesh was 1434 and the government sanctioned these posts of doctors. However, out of 1434 only 985 doctors were posted in tribal areas as on 1 July 1997. The reasons given by the State Government for not posting the sanctioned doctors were remoteness of areas, non-availability of basic facilities and tendency of the doctors to get posted in urban areas.

The Government of India has also failed to take any measures to protect the vital medicinal plants, animals and minerals necessary for the full enjoyment of right to highest attainable standards of health by indigenous peoples.

In an evaluation of Integrated Tribal Development Projects (Study No 166 of 1997), the Programme Evaluation Organisation of the Planning Commission of India stated that most of the schools in TSP areas were lacking teaching staff and in most of the States having TSP areas, the medical facilities were not available up to the mark and about 78 per cent of the sample villages had no Primary Health Centre within a distance of 5 kms.

The misuse, diversion and non-utilisation of funds meant for indigenous and tribal peoples are rampant. The Planning Commission in its Report No. 3 of 1999 reported that "the Assam

Tribal Development Authority spent Rs.4.03 Crore towards purchase of teaching aids for educational institution having 50 per cent or more Scheduled Tribes (ST) students which was earmarked for family oriented income generation schemes for ST population below poverty line. It was further disclosed that the purchase was against Government sanction of Rs.1.50 Crore only. Proper procedure for the purchase was not followed and quotations were called without mention of the specific items". The Planning Commission urged that "such purchases are required to be investigated and responsibility fixed" but no action has been taken.

The issues of availability, accessibility, acceptability and adaptability must be taken into account in the formulation of the programmes for right to education and right to highest attainable standards of health under the Draft National Policy.

The suggestion of the Draft National Policy to "encourage qualified doctors from tribal communities to serve tribal areas" is an attempt to further ghettoize the indigenous peoples. Serving in the rural areas for a period of 10 years with five years exclusively in Tribal Sub-Plan areas must be made mandatory for all government doctors and necessary administrative measures need to be taken. All the vacancies of medical staff in the Tribal Sub-Plan areas need to be filled up within a specified time frame. The government should provide additional benefits to medical staff working in TSP area and concomitant budgetary allocations need to be made under the TSP.

The government needs to promote traditional health care system and all measures be taken for protection of vital medicinal plants, animals and minerals necessary to the full enjoyment of health of indigenous peoples. "Traditional and Alternative Medicinal Act" be adopted with a view to (i) improve the quality and delivery of health care services to the indigenous and tribal peoples through the development of traditional and alternative health care and to integrate it into the national health care delivery system, and (ii) to seek a legally workable basis by which indigenous and tribal societies would own their knowledge of traditional medicine and the government would provide resources to enable the indigenous peoples to design, deliver and control such services so that they may enjoy the highest attainable standard of physical and mental health.

RELIGIOUS VIEWS ON BIRTH CONTROL

Religions vary widely in their views of the ethics of birth control. In Christianity, the Roman Catholic Church accepts only Natural Family Planning, while Protestants maintain a wide range of views from allowing none to very lenient. Views in Judaism range from the stricter Orthodox sect to the more relaxed Reformed sect.

In Islam, contraceptives are allowed if they do not threaten health or lead to sterilty, although their use is discouraged. Hindus may use both natural and artificial contraceptives.

Birth Control Education

Many teenagers, most commonly in developed countries, receive some form of sex education in school. What information should be provided in such programmes is hotly contested, especially in the United States and Great Britain. Possible topics include reproductive anatomy, human sexual behaviour, information on sexually transmitted diseases (STDs), social aspects of sexual interaction, negotiating skills intended to help teens follow through with a decision to remain abstinent or to use birth control during sex, and information on birth control methods.

One type of sex education programme used mainly in the United States is called abstinence-only education, and it promotes sexual abstinence until marriage. The programme does not provide information on birth control, or it heavily emphasises information such as failure rates and strategies for avoiding intimate situations. Advocates of abstinence-only education believe that the programmes will result in decreased rates of teenage pregnancy and STD infection. In an Internet survey of 1,400 women who found and completed a 10-minute multiple-choice online questionnaire listed in one of several popular search engines, women who received sex education from schools providing primarily abstinence information, or contraception and abstinence information equally, reported fewer unplanned pregnancies than those who received primarily contraceptive information, who in turn reported fewer unplanned pregnancies than those who received no information. However, randomised controlled trials demonstrate that abstinence-only sex education programmes increase the rates of pregnancy and STDs in the teenage population. Professional medical organisations, including the AMA, AAP, ACOG, APHA, and Society for Adolescent Medicine, support comprehensive sex education (providing abstinence and contraceptive information) and oppose the sole use of abstinence-only sex education.

Many studies of fertility implicitly equate temporal management, biomedical contraception, and "modernity" on the one hand, and "tradition," the lack of intentional timing, and uncontrolled fertility on the other.

REVIEW OF LITERATURE

1. Breast-feeding patterns and lactational amenorrhoea among the Warli tribals: a socio-anthropological inquiry. Carneiro P, Association for Family Health and Life-India, New Delhi.

Data on breast-feeding patterns and lactational amenorrhoea were collected as part of a socio-anthropological inquiry conducted among the Warli tribals living along the west coast of India. A need to study and length of lactational amenorrhoea among these tribal women arose because in the complete absence of the use of contraception, lactational amenorrhoea acts as a natural birth spacer in this population. Analysis of the data shows that the suckling frequency during lactation, the sex of the child born, and the nutritional status of the women influence the length of lactational amenorrhoea. The consequences of variations in the length of lactational amenorrhoea on other related demographic parameters are also mentioned.

2. Prevalence of female infertility and its socio-economic factors in Tribal communities of Central India, Kumar D, *Rural and Remote Health* 7: 456. (Online), 2007, Available from: http://www.rrh.org.au

The Khairwar tribe of India is dwindling due to infertility and migration. The study investigates an extensive infertility problem among Khairwar and non-Khairwar tribes in the same geographical area. The objective of the study was to determine for the first time the prevalence of infertility in these two tribal groups. The study was undertaken to gain insight into the problem of infertility in the Khairwar tribe. Our study explored the possible association between prevalence of female infertility and some selected socio-economic variables. The observed infertility among Khairwar women was 7.2 per cent, a higher incidence than among non-Khairwar women.

Tribal communities are vulnerable because they are isolated from mainstream resources; and this community does not have easy access to the Indian health delivery system. However the Khairwars do not appear interested in seeking this assistance. Instead, they believe in local traditional healers (gunias). Childless women are particularly vulnerable in their old age in tribal society. Infertility also complicates marital dynamics, sometimes leading to marital instability, and occasionally divorce, polygamy or remarriage. Because motherhood is considered a mandatory status, infertile women may be harassed and tormented. Infertile tribal women suffer most profoundly in their relationship with their in-laws and other community members.

3. Family planning practices among tribals of South Rajasthan, India, Sharma V, Sharma A.

The objective was to examine the practices of family size limitation among tribal people of South Rajasthan and traditional methods of contraception used by them. The study was conducted in 4 tribal blocks of Udaipur District (Badgaon, Girwa, Jhadol [Falasia], and Kherwada), selected by simple random sampling. 250 eligible couples (with wives in the age group 15-44 years) were included. They were analysed with reference to elementary knowledge about modern family planning methods; practice of family planning and contraception; and sexual and child rearing practices.

The couples were interviewed by means of a pre-tested detailed questionnaire. A large number of primitive societies still follow traditional customs of sexual behaviour and child rearing. The methods accepted by them appear to be those that have some monetary incentives attached to them, e.g., vasectomy and tubectomy. There also seemed to be a significant KAP gap or credibility gap between their knowledge and actual practice of contraception. While 60.8 per cent of the couples possessed some knowledge about at least one modern method of contraception, only 19 per cent of them were using a modern method of family planning, and that irregularly. A small percentage were also found to be practicing both traditional and modern methods together (6.8%), while 11.2 per cent of couples relied entirely on traditional methods for limiting family size. In all, about 25.4 per cent of the tribal couples were using some form of family planning. Tribal women also used vaginal douches post-coitally for contraception. A small number of tribal women also described a sort of vaginal sponge soaked in various solutions. The practice of extended breastfeeding was universal among the tribal people. Similarly, the practice of observing total abstinence for certain days of the month and for a period of 2-3 months following delivery also bolstered family planning. PMID: 12346802 [PubMed - indexed for MEDLINE].

4. Ethnomedicinal plants used by the tribals of Simlipal bioreserve, Orissa, India: A pilot study, Kambaska Kumar Behera, Department of Agriculture Biotechnology, Orissa Univesity of Agriculture and Technology (OUAT), Bhubaneswar, Orissa,India, 751003. Email: kambaska@yahoo.co.in

Herbal medicine has been widely practiced throughout the world since ancient times. These medicines are safe and environmentally friendly. According to WHO about 80 per cent of the world's population relies on traditional medicine for their primary health care. India, being one of the world's 12 mega biodiversity countries, enjoys export of herbal raw material worth U.S. $100-114 million per year approximately. Currently the Government of India, realising the value of the country's vast range of medicinal plants, has embarked on a mission of documenting the traditional knowledge about medicinal plants and herbs. This investigation, in a small way, takes up the enumeration of plants with potential medicinal value, which are used by the tribal groups, residing in and around Similipal Bioreserve of Mayurbhanj, Orissa, India. This report elucidates a rich and unique profile of phyto-diversity of the area surveyed, with 89 species belongs to 52 families and 79 genera of medicinal plants.

5. Induced abortion in India, Saseendran Pallikadavath and R William Stones 'Opportunities and Choices' Programme, Southampton Statistical Sciences Research Institute, University of Southampton, Highfield, Southampton SO17 1BJ, UK.

In India study of induced abortion using complete birth history of women using a nationally representative survey is currently lacking. In India son preference is attributed to the rise in the incidence of induced abortion. Research that can provide induced abortion rates and maternal and social correlates can provide better insights in the issue of sex preference and induced abortion apart from providing a complete account of induced abortion for India.

Methods: Complete birth histories of 90,303 ever married women between 15-49 years of age from the 1998-1999 National Family Health Survey were used to compute birth order-specific induced abortion ratios. This involved a great deal of data manipulation using syntax based computations. The influence of maternal and social variables was assessed using logistic regression.

Results: The overall induced abortion ratio was 17.04 per 1,000 pregnancies. The lowest induced abortion ratio was 5.27 per 1,000 pregnancies for first birth order, increased to 25.81 for third birth order and then declined marginally and non-linearly. Education of women was the most important factor that was associated with induced abortion. Having first and second child late was related to previous induced abortion. Living in rural areas substantially reduced the odds of induced abortion. Nationally, sex of the previous child was not significantly associated with induced abortion. Increasing women's education would have profound implications to induced abortions in India. Unplanned and unintended pregnancies rather than sex of the previous child appears to be an important factor associated with induced abortion nationally.

6. Culture, Religion and Reproductive Behaviour in Two Indigenous Communities of Northeastern India: A Discussion of Some Preliminary Findings Udoy Sankar Saikia, Ross Steele and Gour Dasvarma

In spite of enjoying a higher level of female autonomy in a strong matrilineal kinship system, women in matrilineal societies in northeast India have the highest fertility in the country. This direct association of high female autonomy and high fertility challenges the most commonly observed inverse relationship between these two variables in other populations. Preliminary findings from a comparative analysis of the Khasis and the Karbis—two tribal communities with two different kinship systems, highlight the fact that in traditional tribal societies decisions regarding reproduction are not only influenced by individual level factors. Instead, this paper argues that the perceptions and the behaviour related to reproduction are strongly, even predominantly, determined by prevailing cultural and religious values, that form the basis of socially-sanctioned realities in these communities.

It is also argued that reproductive behaviour in these communities is strongly influenced by the insecurities associated with minority-group status. This paper highlights the reality of reproductive norms among these tribal groups and hypothesises that the perception of minority status and the adoption of a more defensive position vis-à-vis outside groups has impacted on fertility outcomes in these communities. This phenomenon calls for further development and refinement of India's National Population Policy.

Based on these preliminary findings this study suggests that social norms and values in the traditional tribal societies wield a stronger influence than individual values in determining the fertility behaviour in those societies. High female autonomy does empower women to take decisions on their own, especially decisions regarding their own health care and reproduction, but this does not necessarily mean that these decisions will be to reduce family size. In an environment with pro-natalist social and cultural norms and a strong traditional society, high female autonomy may encourage women to produce more children. This paper has highlighted the reality of reproductive norms among these tribal groups in an attempt to emphasise the hypothesis that the perception of minority status and the adoption of a more defensive position vis-à-vis outside groups have impacted on fertility outcomes. Proof of this hypothesis would make a most relevant contribution to the Indian Government's attempt to develop population policies more responsive to the needs and aspirations of local ethnic communities.

7. Folk herbal medicines from tribal area of Rajasthan, India, S.S. Katewa , B.L. Chaudhary and Anita Jain, Laboratory of Ethno-botany and Agro-stology, Department of Botany, College of Science, ML Sukhadia University, Udaipur 313 001, India, accepted 8 January 2004.

A floristic survey of ethno-medicinal plants occurring in the tribal area of Rajasthan was conducted to assess the potentiality of plant resources for modern treatments. The information on medicinal uses of plants is based on the exhaustive interviews with local physicians practicing indigenous system of medicine, village headmen, priests and tribal folks. The Aravalli hills of Mewar region of Rajasthan are inhabited by many tribes; Bhil, Garasia, Damor and Kathodia being the main ones. In a floristic survey 61 ethno-medicinal plant species belonging to 38 families were recorded from this region. A categorical list of plant species along with their plant part/s used and the mode of administration reported to be for effective control in different ailments is prepared.

8. Folk herbal medicines used in birth control and sexual diseases by tribals of southern Rajasthan, India, Anita Jain*, S. S. Katewa, B. L. Chaudhary and Praveen Galav, Laboratory of Ethno-botany and Agro-stology, Department of Botany, College of Science, M.L. Sukhadia University, Udaipur 313001, Rajasthan, India, 2003

An ethno-botanical survey of tribal area of southern Rajasthan was carried out during the year 2001-2002 for ethno-sexicological herbal medicines. The information on ethno-sexicological herbs is based on the exhaustive interview with local medicine-men and-women, birth attendants and other knowledgeable persons who prescribe their own herbal preparation to check birth control, including abortion at initial stages, preventing conception or by making either member of the couple sterile and to cure various sexual diseases like leucorrhoea, gonorrhoea, menorrhagia, to regularise menses and syphilis in both the sexes. During ethno-botanical survey, 53 plants belonging to 33 families have been reported from the study area, which are used to cure sexual diseases, and for family planning. A list of plant species along with their local name, habit, flowering and fruiting period, plant part/s used and the mode of administration to cure the sexual diseases are given.

9. Some lesser known oral herbal contraceptives in folk claims as anti-fertility and fertility induced plants in Bastar region of Chhatisgarh, Rajiv Rai, Vijendra Nath, Author Affiliation: Division of Biodiversity and Sustainable Management, Tropical Forest Research Institute, PO. RFRC, Jabalpur 482 021, India. Document Title: Journal of Natural Remedies, 2005 (Vol. 5) (No. 2) 153-159

The traditional knowledge prevailing among Gond tribes of the Bastar region in Chattisgarh, India, regarding the use of various plants as anti-fertility—and fertility-inducing agents was studied and described. The documentation of traditional knowledge from Gond tribes was conducted during ethno-botanical studies. Information was collected by interviewing local vaidyas and traditional herbal healers prevalent in Bastar. They have immense knowledge about plants and drugs being utilised by tribals for the last several centuries by collecting plant parts to prevent birth as oral contraceptives and anti-fertility agents and also as fertility-inducing agents. The lesser known 22 herbal plants used by Gond tribes of Bastar (18 plants as antifertility-inducing agents and 4 as fertility-inducing agents) was briefly described along with botanical and vernacular names, family and methods of preparation of drugs and their dosages. The knowledge of plants used by traditional herbal healers for anti-fertility purposes and isolation of their active ingredients would be of immense help to replace synthetic drugs.

10. Ethno-pharmacology: Knowledge and Use of Medicine among the Santhals of Jharkhand, Supervisor: Prof. P. C. Joshi, Th 15450

Deals with the traditional plant use and management which is an indigenous perception of the natural world, meaning thereby how the specific plant is regarded as sacred, or where a social control determine rights of access to certain areas of land. This will in turn influence how community members behave towards those resources. Similarly, if a disease is believed to be of spiritual rather than natural origin, the remedies used may will posses more symbolic significance than the pharmacological activity. Attempts to understand how Santhal perceive their plant world.

11. Breast-feeding and Infant Feeding Practices in Tribal Areas of India. Bhatnagar S, 1985, Department of Planning and Evaluation, ICMR

Among the selected blocks covered under the study 100 per cent were Hindus in Andhra Pradesh, Madhya Pradesh and Orissa while in Meghalaya and Manipur majority were Christians, in Shellabholeganj PHC 50 per cent were tribals with their own religion which is same form of animism and ancestor worship. Four-fifth of families were nuclear, living under unsatisfactory environmental sanitation using surface water.

Migration is not significant among tribals of Meghalaya, Manipur, Orissa and Andhra Pradesh while tribals from Rajasthan and Madhya Pradesh migrated to far off places in search of livelihood and Garos and Khasis migrated within their own hilly areas in the State only. As many as 88 per cent of pregnant women had no immunisation against T.T and were not given iron and folic acid and 90 per cent no ante-natal check-up.

The place of delivery in case of 89 per cent cases was at home. However, birth attendant was untrained Dai in 50 per cent cases and preference for trained Dai was observed among Halbas (39%) in Madhya Pradesh and for ANM/LHV by Khasis (41%). Most of the children (96.5%) were breast-fed while 59 per cent were breast-fed demand followed by a feeding schedule (13%). However, 53.5 per cent of mothers never cleaned their breast before or while feeding.

Most of the mothers in Andhra Pradesh, Meghalaya and Orissa put the baby to breast milk within 6 hours while in Manipur within 6-12 hours and in Rajasthan and Madhya Pradesh after 2-3 days of birth. Most of tribals viz. Koyas, Lambadis, Rajgonds, Gonds and Halbas and Kamaras fed colostrum 100 per cent, whereas the corresponding percentage of Nogol, Khasis and Khandas was 64, 41 and 44 per cent respectively.

Among the tribal groups who did not feed colostrum to the new-born child Bhils ranked first (98%), followed by Garos (96%) and Santhals (87%). It was found alarming that 33 per cent of tribal group felt that colostrum is not good for baby's stomach. The highest proportions of Koyas, Komars, Rajgonds (100% each). Lambadis (97%), Gonds (85%), Halbas (90%), Nagas (80%) fed colostrum as first diet while among those who fed sweetened water Khasis ranked first (78%), followed by Garos (41%) and Nagas (13%). Thirty six per cent of each of tribal groups felt it to be the customary practice to feed colostrum for cleaning of stomach.

12. Women and Forest: A Study of the Warlis of Western India, Indra Munshi Department of Sociology, University of Mumbai, Publisher: M/s Natural Remedies Private Ltd.

With the loss of access to forests, the Warlis have been deprived not only of an important source of livelihood, but also the basis of their religion and culture. This has affected women and men in different ways. Changes in the forest management system, and the accompanying socio-cultural transformation of the Warli community, have reduced Warli women's access to land and forest. This has exacerbated the traditional tension between the two genders, which is manifest in a renewed wave of witch hunting. Witch hunting may also be explained as an attack on the high status of women in the past and the change in social relations in favour of men. Nevertheless, the Warli women are taking on the combined might of patriarchy and the men within their community as part of their fight to pre serve forests.

13. Kapoor, A. K.; Kshatriya, Gautam K. "Fertility and mortality differentials among selected tribal population groups of north-western and eastern India".

Selection potential based on differential fertility and mortality has been computed for six tribal groups inhabiting different geo-climatic conditions, namely: Sahariya, Mina and Bhil of the State of Rajasthan, north-western India, and Munda, Santal and Lodha of the State of West Bengal, eastern India. Irrespective of the methodology, the total index of selection was found to be highest among Lodhas, followed by Sahariyas, Santals, Bhils, Mundas and Minas. Incidently, Lodha and Sahariya are two of the seventy-four notified primitive tribal groups of India, and these two study populations show the highest index of total selection, mainly because of a higher embryonic and post-natal mortality. The relative contribution of the fertility component to the index of total selection is higher than the corresponding mortality component in all tribal groups. The analysis of post-natal mortality components indicates that childhood mortality constitutes the bulk of post-natal mortality, suggesting that children under 5 years need better health care in these tribal groups.

14. Nath, Dilip C.; Leonetti, Donna L.; Steele, Matthew S. "Analysis of birth intervals in a non-contracepting Indian population: An evolutionary ecological approach

Reproductive strategies are related to ecological constraints. This paper examines data on early birth spacing in a scheduled caste, Bengali-speaking, non-contracepting population of the Karimganj district of southern Assam, India, taking an evolutionary ecological perspective. It is found that on average birth intervals closed by boy-boy are longer than those closed by girl-girl. Birth spacing tends to be longer among upper-income and Craftsman sub-caste mothers. The presence of a 'grandmother' in the household shortens spacing. These findings are compatible with an evolutionary-based reproductive decision-making process.

15. Anna Glasier Lothian Primary Care NHS Trust and University of Edinburgh Department of Reproduction and Development, Edinburgh, EH4 1NL, Scotland email: a.glasier@ed.ac.uk, Published online: 01 October 2002 | doi:10.1038/ncb-nm-fertilitys3

16. Bajpai S and Sadgopal M, eds (1996). *Her Healing Heritage*. Ahmedabad/Coimbatore: CHETNA/LSPSS

This book is based on the 12-State study of local health traditions relating to mother and child health conducted by Lok Swasthya Parampara Samvardhan Samithi based in Coimbatore and CHETNA, Ahmedabad. It has a section on the Dai Tradition. Only circumstantial evidence of placental stimulation is recorded, as the surveyors were not aware of these practices. The indigenous midwifery traditions in South Asia include the practice of reviving a limp newborn by stimulating the placenta. From our collection of personal observations and references in literature, we know that such treatment of the placenta (with the umbilical cord still uncut) is widespread in India. It has also been identified in Bangladesh and in Burma. The methods of stimulating the placenta vary from place to place, using wet or dry heat, manual pressure and occasionally application of certain substances. In India the midwives who do it explain that the *jeeva* or 'life force' (or *praan*, *jaan*, etc.) is contained in the placenta. They say that if a baby doesn't breathe or cry at once and appears lifeless they can bring life into its body in this way.

STATEMENT OF THE PROBLEM

According 2001 census the total tribal population of India is 84 million, amounting to 8.85 per cent to the country's total population. According to the Anthropological Survey of India, there are 750 tribes in the country. Out of the 750 tribes, the Ministry of Tribal Affairs, Government of India has classified 698 groups as Scheduled Tribes. Out of the 698 groups, 75 tribes have been declared as primitive tribes.

Each of the above mentioned tribe has its own dialect, cultural life style and ethno medical beliefs and practices. "Medical world of tribals – explorations illness, ideology, body symbolism and ritual, a book by Tribhuwan Robin is a classic example. In his book Dr. Tribhuwan has shown how different is the medical world view of tribe as compared to the scientific rationale of medicine, disease, body image and therapies. The research problem we have posed here is that considering the ethno-medical beliefs and practices, the cultural life styles, the educational level, ecology in which the tribes live in, their health behaviour and the way they view the concept of body image, birth control and contraceptive practices from an emic (insider's) perspective needs to be understood, before drawing health education and birth control strategy from an etic (outsider's) perspective.

Secondly, each tribal culture has its distinct beliefs about health and disease, which means the strategies for birth control and contraceptives need to be planned is such a way that they are accepted by the tribe concerned. Thirdly, what efforts are made by the Tribal Research and Training Institutes as well as the Health Departments in the country to document the birth-control and contraceptive practices of the tribes of this country, so as to draft culturally acceptable and appropriate strategies?

Fourthly, given to understand that tribal people have their own world view about medicine, body image, human reproduction, birth control and contraceptives, how useful is the rationale of health education, birth control and contraception which has its roots in modern medicine?

Lastly, is any thought given to researches that have pointed out the reactions of tribal people to modern or allopathic strategies of birth control and contraceptives.

In their book captioned "mirage of health and development", Jain N.S and Tribhuwan Robin (1996:232) revealed the specific contraceptive practices among the Korkus. There study showed that Korkus have their own perceptions about natural spacing and contraceptive practices. The study revealed that the Korkus were not aware of the significance of the use of modern contraceptives. They were reluctant to use oral pills and IUD and felt that:

- Copper T insertion leads to tearing of uterus;
- It hurts the penis of males during sexual intercourse;
- Causes pain in the lower abdomen and back as well;
- Its insertion gives rise to bleeding and white discharge;
- It decreases the breast milk of the mother.

Similarly most of the Korku women interviewed said that consumption of oral pills made a woman's abdominal region fat.

The perception of the males regarding the condoms, the study revealed that males do not get sexual satisfaction because of the use of condoms. Secondly, the men have the problem of storing condom packets in the house and disposing them. Some Korku males shared the fear that our children may see the condom packets and start asking questions.

Given the above background of the research problem as well as review of literature, some of the research questions that cropped up through the study were as follows:

RESEARCH QUESTIONS

- To what extent are agencies providing health and educational services as well as the Tribal Research Training Institutes documenting indigenous knowledge and practices of birth control and contraceptives among tribes of India?
- Are any efforts made to scientifically analyse the ingredients of plants, animals, mineral resources used by the tribals for birth control, so as to check on their safety and efficacy?
- What is the scientific rationale of the tribal beliefs and practices of birth control?
- How can the traditional medical practitioners be involved in birth control and contraceptive campaigns/ programmes in tribal areas?
- What strategies should be evolved to involve social and health scientists in birth control and contraceptive campaigns?

OBJECTIVES OF THE STUDY

- To understand the concept of body image, human reproduction, birth control and contraception from traditional and modern perspectives;
- To study the policies of WHO and the Government of India regarding birth control and contraception;
- To document the concept of medicine, body image, human reproduction process, birth control and contraceptives among selected tribes of India;
- To analyse and clarify common or universal practices of birth control and contraceptives among the tribes studied;
- To develop a theoretical model for studying traditional beliefs and practices regarding body image, reproductive health, birth control and contraception;

- To suggest recommendation to policy makers about birth control and contraceptive campaign strategies in tribal areas.

SIGNIFICANCE OF THE STUDY

People everywhere act on the basis of knowledge and beliefs about the world, about themselves and about action itself. Beliefs form among every people a system: this system can be seen as a group of propositions about the world, which on further examination, reveal themselves to be ordered in their relationships with one another.

Hallowell I.A. (1942) has rightly pointed out that human beings live in a meaningful universe not a world of bare physical objects. Social life thus, has meaning, the things people do are communicable and this entails a system of signs and symbols in which the meaning is embedded and expressed.

At the theoretical level this study aims to show how tribal beliefs and practices regarding body image, reproductive health, birth control and contraceptive practices are deeply rooted in their culture. That these practices are built on their rationale of body image, reproductive health, birth control, contraceptive practices and the medical resources they have been using since time immemorial.

The data presented and interpreted in this book will certainly help social, health and medical scientists, pharmacologists, ethno-botanists etc to develop new theoretical insights in their respective disciplines. At the more practical level research scholars can take up tribe wise studies to analyse and explore the safety, efficacy and wider applications of tribal practices about birth control and contraceptives.

This study will be an eye opener for the government departments working in the field of Tribal Development, Health, Health Education, Social Forestry and I.C.D.S. etc to plan, implement, monitor and follow-up natural resource management programmes so as to preserve tribal knowledge and the medical resources they know of. NGO's working in developing medical resources among tribal peoples will also be benefited from this study.

2

Research Methodology

BACKGROUND OF THE STUDY

Both, Dr. Robin D.Tribbuwan and Dr. Benazir Patil have worked independently on health and medical issues of tribal, rural and slum societies. Dr. Tribhuwan has published several papers, books and manuals on tribal health, medicine, nutrition and health care, while Dr. Patil is an expert on health policies.

While pursuing his doctoral and post doctoral research Dr. Tribhuwan came across several concepts among tribals in the field of body image, birth control and reproduction, which had some scientific sense, as well as some practices were superstitious and illogical. These aspects were discussed by Dr. Robin with Dr. Benazir who too worked among the Santhals of Orissa in this area. These discussions and deliberations among the authors of this book resulted into development of research tools to document tribal perceptions of body image, human reproduction and birth control by the authors. Thus, five tribes namely Thakars, Santhals, Gonds, Nagas and Mavchis were selected to study the above mentioned concepts. The research methodology for the project is as follows:

LOCALE OF THE STUDY

The present study was conducted is Maharashtra, Nagaland, Orissa, Jharkhand and Chattisgrah in selected tribal hamlets of the above mentioned tribes. The researchers developed good rapport with the medical practitioners, elderly people, the functionaries, pregnant and lactating women so as to gather relevant data.

TARGET POPULATION

The Target population of the study are Nagas, Gonds, Santhals, Thakars and Mavchis. The authors targeted traditional medical practitioners, pregnant and lactating mothers, elderly women, and health care providers etc to gather relevant data.

DATA COLLECTION

Both secondary and primary data was collected by the authors:

(a) ***Secondary Data:*** An effect was made by the authors to search books, magazines, articles and internet to gather secondary data published by various authors with regard to body image, reproductive health systems, birth control and contraception among tribals. Material obtained books, journals, magazines, and other sources, which is duly acknowledged by the authors;

(b) ***Primary Data:*** An interview guide was prepared after a pilot study is one tribal village. It was tested in another tribe, modified and finalised for gathering relevant data. Indepth interviews of key informants such as: traditional medical practitioners including shamans, herbalists, bone setters and more importantly traditional birth attendants; pregnant and lactating mothers; elderly women; staff from government primary health centre and private clinic staff was interviewed. 50 respondents inclusive of the entire above category were interviewed from each tribe and the region. Thus, besides this, focus group discussions, participatory debates etc were held so as to validate the data. Participatory observation method was yet another tool used by the researchers.

DATA ANALYSIS

Since the data was qualitative in nature, it was analysed manually.

SAMPLING PROCEDURES

Purposive sampling procedure was adopted to select the sample because of the qualitative nature of the data.

CHAPTER SCHEME

The data gathered, analysed and interpreted from primary and secondary sources is presented in eight chapters. These are as follows:

(i) Chapter One

Medicine, Birth-control and Contraceptive Practices—Traditional and Modern Perspective

In this chapter the authors have presented basic concepts and definitions of medicine, birth-control and contraceptive practices prevalent in both traditional as well as modern era. This chapter also presents the research problem, research questions, objectives and significance of the study, including review of literature under this area.

(ii) Chapter Two

Research Methodology

As the name of the chapter suggests, the research methodology used by authors to collect, analyse, interpret and present primary and secondary data is given in this chapter.

(iii) Chapter Three

Body Image and Human Reproduction Process

Chapter three throws light on the tribal as well as modern concept of body image and human reproduction process. On one hand allopathy is proven, factual and validated scientifically through research, whereas the tribal medical systems associate the concept of body image and human reproduction on the basis of indigenous medical knowledge developed within their cultures by elites and medical practitioners, which is based more on trial and error methods and lacks scientific validation. Thus chapter three sets the stage for findings and discussions reported in subsequent chapters.

(iv) Chapter Four

Body Image, Human Reproduction and Birth Control Practices Among Thakars

Thakars are one of the major tribes in Maharashtra state, found in six to seven districts, this tribe is extensively researched by Dr. Tribhuwan for over fifteen years. Due to the close rapport with the Thakars, the information reported in this chapter is holistic and presents their concepts about disease etiology, body symbolism, nature and role of medical practitioners, traditional contraceptive practices etc from an insider's perspective.

(v) Chapter Five

Ethno-medical Therapies for Contraception and Impotency Among Santhals

Like the earlier chapter, this chapter also presents a brief ethnographic background of Santhals of Orissa, with an emphasis on some of the therapies used by the tribe for impotency, abortion, contraception, treatment of menstrual disorders, lactation amenorrhoea etc.

(vi) Chapter Six

Ethno-medical Practices Among the Gonds

Chapter six highlights the ethno-medical practices among the Gonds of Chattisgarh with specific focus on practices and methods inducing abortions and impotency curative practices.

(vii) Chapter Seven

Maternal Health and Birth Control Practices of Mavchi Tribe

Chapter seven presents the MCH and birth control practices among the Mavchis of Mandurbar.

(viii) Chapter Eight

Body Image, Reproduction and Birth Control Practices Among the Ao Nagas

The chapter on Ao-Nagas emphasises on their ethno-medical beliefs and practices including their perceptions on birth control and body image. The chapter also reveals that impact of Christianity and modernisation on the Ao-Naga culture has influenced their traditional practices regarding the above subject to a great extent.

As the title suggests this chapter focusses on the above issues.

(ix) Chapter Nine

Summary, Conclusions and Recommendations

As the name suggests this chapter presents conclusions and lays down emphasis on the need to seriously and scientifically look into the area of birth control, reproduction, contraception among the tribals of India, so as to provide them appropriate and culturally acceptable health care and educational programmes in this area. The recommendations given by the authors to the policy makers as well as health care providers will certainly contribute in improving present system of health care delivery in this area.

3

Body Image and Human Reproduction Process

The chapter is divided into two parts, section one talks about the scientific concepts regarding the human reproduction process, whereas section two deals with the perceptions of tribals and their conceptual understanding about the human body and the reproduction process.

SECTION ONE

CONCEPTION: BIOLOGICAL PROCESS

For a couple to conceive, several biological processes need to take place successfully and at the right time. During her menstrual cycle, a woman's hormones stimulate the growth, maturation, and release of an egg from her ovary. This process begins when the hypothalamus signals the pituitary gland to send a hormone known as follicle-stimulating hormone (FSH) to the ovaries, prompting them to prepare an egg for ovulation. The FSH stimulates a group of follicles to grow on the surface of the ovary.

Over the next two weeks (the follicular phase of the cycle), the eggs mature and levels of estrogen, which is produced by the ovaries, increase. As the estrogen levels increase, the pituitary gland decreases its production of FSH, and LH (luteinising hormone) production is then triggered. The cervix begins to produce fertile alkaline mucus to help keep potential sperm alive and to speed their transport.

The LH production peaks, signaling the ovary to release a mature egg (usually only one) from its follicle in a process known as ovulation. The egg enters and begins to travel through the fallopian tube. The egg remains viable for about 24 hours. For fertilisation to occur, a sperm must locate and penetrate the awaiting egg while it is in the fallopian tube. If fertilisation occurs, the fertilised egg, or embryo, continues to travel down the fallopian tube into the uterus.

On approximately the seventh day following fertilisation, the embryo develops chorionic villi, which are special protrusions on its surface that enable it to attach, or implant, in the lining of the uterus. The chorionic villi produce a hormone called human chorionic gonadotropin (hCG) that signals the corpus luteum to continue to increase in size and produce more progesterone to maintain the pregnancy; hCG is the hormone that is picked up by a pregnancy testing kit.

Thus in order for a couple to conceive, both the male and female reproductive systems must be functioning properly.

For a woman this means:

- Ovulation occurs and leads to the production of a viable egg;
- The fallopian tubes are open and functioning properly to allow the egg and sperm to meet;
- The woman's vagina, cervix uterus, and fallopian tubes allow for the sperm to travel to the fallopian tube and attempt to locate the egg;
- The fertilised egg is able to move into the uterus and is not blocked from implanting in the wall of the uterus.

For a man this means:

- The testes produce viable, or normal sperm, as well as testosterone, the male hormone;
- Sexual intercourse involving an erection and ejaculation must occur during the woman's fertile period;

- Ejaculation is normal, with semen going through the man's urethra into the vagina;
- The sperm that are produced are properly shaped, able to move rapidly, and able to find the fallopian tubes to locate and fertilise the egg.

The pituitary gland and the hypothalamus act as a unit, regulating the activity of most of the other endocrine glands. The pituitary gland lies below the hypothalamus in the hypophyseal fossa of the sphenoid bone. It is connected to the hypothalamus by a stalk. Pituitary gland weighs about 4gm and consists of three distinct parts—The adenohypophysis (anterior lobe), the neurohypophysis (posterior lobe) and between these lobes there is a thin strip of tissue called the intermediate lobe.

Adenohypophysis (anterior lobe): Some of the hormones secreted by the anterior lobe stimulate or inhibit secretion by other endocrine glands (target glands). Other hormones have direct effect on target glands. Following table shows the main relationship between the hypothalamus, the adenohypophysis and the target gland.

Hypothalamus	*Adenohypophysis*	*Target gland or Tissue*
Growth hormone releasing hormone (GHRH)	Growth hormone (GH)	All tissues
Growth hormone release inhibiting hormone (GHRIH) Somatostatin	GH inhibition	All tissue, thyroid gland, islets of Langerhans
Thyroid releasing hormone (TRH)	Thyroid stimulating hormone (TSH)	Thyroid gland
Corticotrophin releasing hormone (CRH)	Adrenocorticotropic hormone	Adrenal cortex
None	Prolactin	Breast
Prolactin inhibiting factor (PIF)	PRL inhibition	Breast
Luteinising hormone releasing hormone (LHRH)	Follicle stimulating hormone	Ovaries and testes
Gonadotropin releasing hormone (GnRH)	Luteinising hormone (LH)	Ovaries and testes

The release of anterior pituitary hormones follows stimulation of the gland by the hormones (releasing hormones) produced by the hypothalamus. Releasing hormones reach pituitary gland through the pituitary portal system of blood vessels. When there is a low level of a target gland hormone, hypothalamus produces the appropriate releasing hormone. The releasing hormone stimulates release of hormone by the anterior pituitary and this in turn stimulates the target gland to produce and release its hormone. When blood level of target gland hormone is increased, it inhibits the secretion of releasing hormone by the hypothalamus.

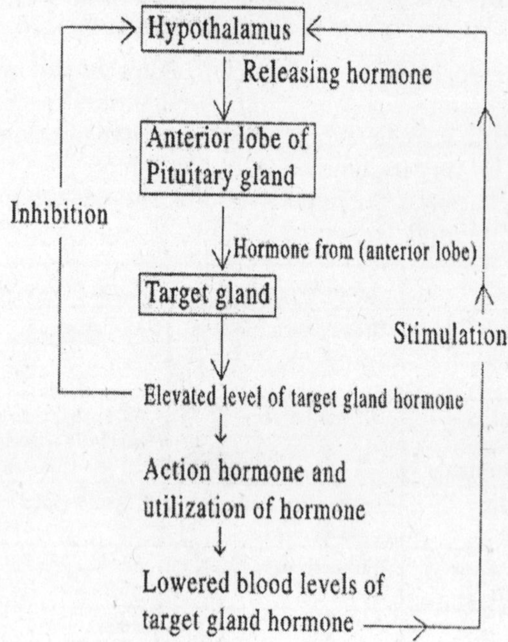

ROLE OF HORMONES IN REPRODUCTION PROCESS

If you are having trouble getting pregnant, it may have something to do with your hormones. Hormones are special chemicals secreted by the glands in your body; they work on specific body parts in order to ensure proper functioning.

Ovulation and menstruation are both triggered by hormone secretion. As a result, infertility is often caused by an imbalance in these hormones. Specifically, the hormone prolactin plays a large role in preventing some women from becoming pregnant.

Prolactin is a chemical that is secreted by your pituitary gland. This is the pea-sized gland found in the middle of your brain, which is responsible for triggering many of your body's processes. Prolactin is found in both men and women and is released at various times throughout the day and night. Prolactin is generally released in order to stimulate milk production in pregnant women. It also enlarges a woman's mammary glands in order to allow her to prepare for breastfeeding.

Hormones that Affect Prolactin

Like many of your body's other processes, the release of prolactin is actually triggered by other hormones. Hormones affecting prolactin include dopamine, serotonin, and thyroid-producing hormone. Serotonin and thyroid hormone help to increase prolactin release, whereas dopamine works to block prolactin release.

Prolactin Changes during Pregnancy

When you are pregnant, prolactin changes are completely normal. In fact, your prolactin must increase in order to encourage the production of milk in your mammary glands. During pregnancy your hormones are all over the place. In particular, your estrogen levels begin to rise, and this is what stimulates the increase in your prolactin levels. After birth, as your baby breastfeeds, nipple stimulation will trigger a further increase in prolactin. Prolactin is what allows you to continue breastfeeding for an extended period of time.

Prolactin and Infertility

Prolactin doesn't just cause your body to increase milk production—it also affects your ovulation and menstrual cycles. This is why it is nearly impossible to become pregnant when you are breastfeeding. (In fact, prolactin is 90 per cent effective against pregnancy in the first months after birth).

Prolactin inhibits two hormones necessary to your ovulation: follicle stimulating hormone (FSH) and gonadotropin releasing hormone (GnRH). Both of these hormones are responsible for helping your eggs to develop and mature in the ovaries, so that they can be released during ovulation. When you have excess prolactin in your bloodstream, ovulation is not triggered, and you will be unable to become pregnant. Prolactin may also affect your menstrual cycle and the regularity of your periods.

Prolactin Irregularities

If you are having difficulties becoming pregnant, it may be due to an irregularity in your prolactin levels. If your have elevated prolactin, this can inhibit ovulation and menstruation. Prolactin levels can be determined through a simple blood test. Normal prolactin levels in women are somewhere between 30 and 600 mIU/I. If your levels measure towards the high end of this spectrum or above, you may be suffering from a prolactin irregularity.

Types of Irregularities

There are two main types of prolactin irregularities. It is possible to suffer from both at one time:

Galactorrhea: this is a condition in which you begin to produce milk spontaneously, without being pregnant or having given birth recently. It is a result of high prolactic levels. Other symptoms include enlarged breasts, painful or tender breasts, irregular menstruation, loss of sex drive and infertility.

Hyperprolactinemia: this literally means too much prolactin in the blood. If you have Hyperprolactinemia, you may also have Galactorrhea, though this is not always the case. Symptoms of high prolactin levels include prolactin levels at or above 600 mIU/I, infertility, irregular menstruation, headache, reduced sex drive and vision problems.

Causes of High Prolactin Levels

There are a few things that may be responsible for your prolactin irregularities. In order to treat your infertility, you will need to determine what is at the bottom of your elevated prolactin levels.

Prolactinoma: this is one of the more common causes of prolactin-induced infertility. Prolactinoma causes a tumour to grow on your pituitary gland. This tumour secretes excess prolactin into your body. About 10 per cent of the population have these tumours. They usually do not pose any health risks, besides infertility, though sometimes they can interfere with vision.

Prescription Drugs

Prescription drugs can cause excess secretion of prolactin. Some anti-depressants, painkillers, and opiates block dopamine, preventing prolactin secretion from being inhibited. This can cause your prolactin levels to rise.

Other Causes

Other more rare causes of prolactin irregularities include thyroid disease, *Polycystic Ovarian Syndrome* (PCOS) and shingles.

The changes in hormone levels in pregnant women are truly profound. Most men find it difficult to fully comprehend what is causing all these changes from mood-swings to constipation, extra sleep to food cravings.

Quite simply, it is the effect of various hormones that is the main contributor to these changes in your partner, but more than that, it's these very same hormone changes that enable her to carry the baby for nine months and assist it to develop.

In a previous article, we discussed in detail the role of the vital hormone b-HCG (beta Human Chorionic Gonadotropin hormone) during pregnancy, then in another issue we discussed the effects of the hormones produced in the pituitary gland, LH (lutenising hormone) and FSH (Follicle Stimulating Hormone) during the ovulation process.

This new piece expands the subject to cover progesterone and estrogens (oestrogen), as well as some other lesser well known hormones. The precise intricate interactions between all of the various hormones swimming around her body is still to be fully explained, however, a large part of the main functions of each hormone is understood and research is continuing on mapping out the full picture.

Progesterone is found in relatively low levels for the first part of a woman's menstrual cycle. It is produced by cells within the ovaries called "granulosa cells" which surround the tiny follicles that will mature to become ovulated eggs.

After ovulation, the "yellow body" (corpus luteum) that released the mature egg into the fallopian tube begins to secrete high levels of progesterone from the granulosa cells within it. This hormone stimulates the growth of rich blood vessels that supply the uterus lining (endometrium). It also causes the expansion of tiny glands in the endometrium that produce a fluid (uterine fluid) that can be used to nourish sperms and embryos that find their way into the uterus. These tiny glands are created by the estrogens hormone and the progesterone takes over the job of making them mature into "feeding structures".

The production of progesterone will normally drop away after about 10 days beyond ovulation. It is this sudden reduction in the hormone that will prompt the menstruation period to begin due to the reduced oxygen supply from the blood vessels that were previously encouraged to grow by the progesterone hormone.

If however, the released egg is fertilised and manages to embed itself into the uterine wall, then the hormone b-HCG is released from the developing placenta, which has the effect of telling the "yellow body" to continue to produce both progesterone and oestrogen. This in turn prevents the start of the menstrual cycle and stops further eggs from being released.

The ovaries continue to produce progesterone (and oestrogen) during the first 8 to 9 weeks until the placenta begins to reduce the amount of b-HCG secreted, which is a signal to the "yellow body" that it is capable of producing these hormones for itself and requires less help.

The Role of Progesterone

The placenta continues to produce both progesterone and oestrogen for the duration of the pregnancy and the levels get higher and higher right up to just before the birth.

The following chart shows the average growth in the level of progesterone within the body during a pregnancy. The dotted line shows what would happen if no fertilisation happened during normal menstrual cycles.

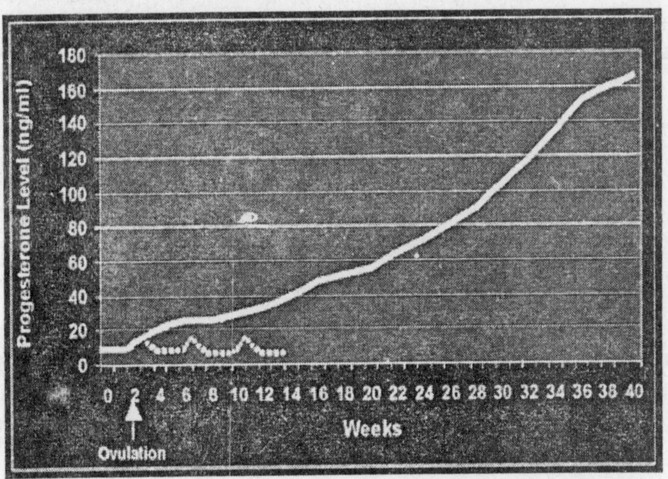

During the pregnancy, the progesterone is needed in the following ways, (mostly in conjunction with oestrogen):

- Makes the endometrium develop and secrete fluids after being primed by estrogen;
- Maintains the functions of the placenta and fights off unwanted cells near the womb that could cause damage to the placenta or foetus;
- Keeps the endometrium in a thickened condition;
- Stops the uterus making spontaneous movements;
- Stimulates the growth of breast tissue;
- Prevents lactation until after the birth (with estrogen);

- Strengthens the mucus plug covering the cervix to prevent infection;
- Strengthens the pelvic walls in preparation for labour;
- Stops the uterus from contracting (thus keeping the baby where it is).

At the end of the pregnancy, the levels of progesterone secreted by the placenta drop off. It is this action that stimulates the beginning of the contractions that will lead to birth. The effects on a woman due to raised levels of progesterone can include any or all of the following:

- Constipation
- Heartburn
- Runny and irritable nose
- Eyesight problems (blurring or headaches)
- Increased kidney infection risk.

A minimum level of about 10ng/ml is required to sustain a pregnancy through the very early stages. It is because of this that doctors can measure the levels of progesterone in the blood to assist in the diagnosis of abnormal pregnancies such as ectopic pregnancy.

Supplements of natural progesterone are sometimes prescribed as a fertility treatment or to assist in reducing the risk of miscarriage. This is found in the form of a cream that is rubbed into the abdomen and thighs or else it arrives as a vaginal suppository or an injection (tablets don't work very well).

The Role of Estrogen (Oestrogen)

Estrogen is the name given to a family of ovarian hormones which all have similar characteristics. During the female menstruation cycle, the production of oestrogen is controlled by the hormone LH (Leutenising Hormone) both indirectly and directly. The "Yellow Body" (corpus luteum) is directly stimulated by LH to produce oestrogen, whereas before ovulation, the granulosa cells of the follicle are stimulated to produce oestrogen via an enzyme called aromatase.

As with progesterone, oestrogen is produced by the placenta throughout a pregnancy and the levels increase steadily until birth. Each hormone plays a vital and complex role during a pregnancy and many of them interact with each other to stimulate various parts of the process.

One role of oestrogen during pregnancy is to regulate the production of progesterone over the full term. As oestrogen is produced by the placenta, progesterone production is stimulated and regulated. Apart from this, oestrogen plays a very important role in the development of the foetus. Without oestrogen, the lungs, kidneys, liver, adrenal glands and other organs would never be triggered into maturation. In fact, the placenta itself would never grow and operate properly if not for oestrogen.

The following list shows some other known jobs undertaken by oestrogen:

- Triggers the maturation of reproductive organs
- Help in the development of sexual characteristics
- Assists in the lactation process
- Regulates bone density in a foetus
- Maintains the endometrium during pregnancy
- Promotes blood flow within the uterus
- Maintains, regulates and triggers the production of other hormones
- Protects female foetuses from the effects of androgens in the mother's system. (Androgens are substances that have a masculinising effect).

The main external effect on women of the increased levels of oestrogen during a pregnancy is the appearance of rashes or red blotches on the skin. It is this effect that is often described as the 'glow' of pregnancy.

Summary of the Other Hormones

The following list gives a quick summary of the primary function of the other pregnancy hormones that have not been discussed up to now:

HSC (Human Chorionic Somatomammotropin)) or HPL (Human Placental Lactogen) This hormone is regulated by estrogen and is produced within the placenta. It plays a part in the development of the foetus and helps the breasts develop the glands that will be required for breastfeeding. It also reduces the level of glucose consumed by the mother. The levels increase steadily from 3 weeks gestation to a limit in the last month of pregnancy.

Calcitonin: This protein based hormone is used to regulate the bone development and to stop calcium from transferring from the bones into the blood system.

Thyroxine (T4 and T3): This is needed for the development of the central nervous system. It also increases oxygen consumption and develops the ability of the foetus to metabolise proteins and carbohydrates. On top of this, it interacts with growth hormones to regulate and stimulate the baby's growth.

Insulin: Helps the baby to store food in it's body and to regulate glucose levels.

Relaxin: Encourages the cervix and the pelvic muscles to relax, thus helping with labour and birth.

Oxytocin: This hormone is released as a response to stretching the cervix or stimulation of the nipples. It has the effect of making the uterus contract so that birth happens rapidly. It also stimulates the mammary glands to produce milk. High levels of progesterone will prevent oxytocin from having an effect. Only when progesterone levels drop close to the birth will the effects of this hormone be felt.

Erythropoietin: Produced in the kidneys, this hormone looks after bone marrow and red blood cell production.

Cortisol: Helps the baby use various foods properly within the body.

Prolactin: This hormone is made by the baby's kidneys and is reduced about a week after birth. The levels remain high within the mother's blood for about two weeks after birth. Prolactin is important for the regulation of the mother's metabolism during the pregnancy and assists in the stimulation of immune system cell growth. It helps prepares the breasts for breastfeeding and promotes the growth of the baby.

DIFFERENT STAGES OF GROWTH

The process leading up to the birth of a newborn baby can be divided into many steps:

About 1 month before conception: Almost all adult males produce thousands of spermatozoa (male germ cells) each second. It would take about 500 of them lined up in a row to total 1 inch in length. They take a month or so to travel from a testicle, through a long tube called the "vas deferens," to reach a small reservoir inside the man's prostate gland. Here, semen (a mixture of spermatozoa and various fluids) is formed. Each spermatozoon contains human DNA. They certainly appear to be living organisms. As seen in a microscope, they seem to be moving energetically with the sole motivation of fusing with an ovum. Most people consider them to be a form of human life, because they appear alive and contain human DNA. Some scientists define "life" so strictly that spermatozoon is not considered alive. Its movements are due to chemical reactions.

Perhaps one day before conception: The woman ovulates and produces one mature ovum (egg cell). It travels down one of her fallopian tubes towards her uterus. It is about 1/100" in diameter, and is barely visible to the naked eye. It also considered by most of the public to be a form of human life, for the above reasons. But it does not meet some scientists' strict definition of a living organism, because it lacks one factor: the ability by itself to reproduce. It can only reproduce with the assistance of a spermatozoon. Some of these scientists have described an ovum as an *"inert globule of organic matter."* It does carry a cargo of human DNA.

At conception: One very lucky spermatozoon out of hundreds of millions ejaculated by the man will penetrate the outside layer of the ovum and fertilise it. This happens typically in the outer third of one of the woman's fallopian tubes. The surface of the ovum changes its electrical characteristics and normally prevents additional sperm from entering. A genetically unique entity is formed shortly thereafter, called a zygote. This is commonly referred to as a *"fertilised ovum."* However that term is not really valid because the ovum ceases to exist after conception. Half of the zygote's 46 chromosomes come from the egg's 23 chromosomes and the other half from the spermatozoon's 23. It has a unique DNA structure, different from that of the ovum and the spermatozoon. The zygote *"is biologically alive. It fulfils the four criteria needed to establish biological life: metabolism, growth, reaction to stimuli, and reproduction."*. It can reproduce itself through twinning at any time up to about 14 days after conception; this is how identical twins are caused.

Conception is the point that most, or all, pro-life groups and conservative Christians define as the beginning of pregnancy. Most of these groups define the start of a human person as occurring at conception. The medical definition of the start of pregnancy is about 10 days later, at implantation. The zygote divides into two cells, called blastomeres. They subdivide once every 12 to 20 hours as the zygote slowly passes down the fallopian tubes.

About 3 days after conception: The zygote now consists of 16 cells and is called a 16 cell morula (pre-embryo). It has normally reached the junction of the fallopian tube and the uterus.

5 days or so after conception: A cavity appears in the center of the morula. The grouping of cells are now called a blastocyst. It has an inner group of cells which will become the fetus and later the newborn; it has an outer shell of cells which will *"become the membranes that nourish and protect the inner group of cells."* It has travelled down the fallopian tubes and has started to attach itself to the endometrium, the inside wall of the uterus (a.k.a. womb). The cells in the inside of the blastocyst, called the embryoblast, start forming the embryo. The outer cells, called the trophoblast, start to form the placenta. It continues to be referred to as a pre-embryo.

9 or 10 days after conception: The blastocyst has fully attached itself to endometrium. Primitive placental blood circulation has begun. This blastocyst has become one of the lucky ones. Most never make it this far in the process.

12 days or so after conception: The blastocyst has started to produce hormones which can be detected in the woman's urine. This is is the event that all (or almost) all pro-choice groups and almost all physicians (who are not conservative Christians) define to be the start of pregnancy. If instructions are followed exactly, a home-pregnancy test may reliably detect pregnancy at this point, or shortly thereafter.

13 or 14 days after conception: A *"primitive streak"* appears. It will later develop into the fetus' central nervous system. This is the point at which spontaneous division of the blastocyst — an event that sometimes generates identical twins — is not longer possible. The pre-embryo is now referred to as an embryo. It is a very small blob of undifferentiated tissue at this stage of development.

3 weeks: The embryo is now about 1/12" long, the size of a pencil point. It most closely resembles a worm—long and thin and with a segmented end. Its heart begins to beat about 18 to 21 days after conception. Before this time, the woman might have noticed that her menstrual period is late; she might suspect that she is pregnant and conduct a pregnancy test. If it is an unwanted pregnancy, she might have already arranged and carried through with an abortion.

4 weeks: The embryo is now about 1/5" long. It looks something like a tadpole. The structure that will develop into a head is visible, as is a noticeable tail. The embryo has structures like the gills of a fish in the area that will later develop into a throat.

5 weeks: Tiny arm and leg buds have formed. Hands with webs between the fingers have formed at the end of the arm buds. Fingerprints are detectable. The face *"has a distinctly reptilian aspect." "...the embryo still has a tail and cannot be distinguished from pig, rabbit, elephant, or chick embryo."*

6 weeks: The embryo is about 1/2" long. The face has two eyes on each side of its head; the front of the face has *"connected slits where the mouth and nose eventually will be."*

7 weeks: The embryo has almost lost its tail. *"The face is mammalian but somewhat pig-like."* Pain sensors appear. Many conservative Christians believe that the embryo can feel pain. However, the higher functions of the brain have yet to develop, and the pathways to transfer pain signals from the pain sensors to the brain have not developed at this time.

2 months: The embryo's face resembles that of a primate but is not fully human in appearance. Some of the brain begins to form; this is the primitive *"reptilian brain"* that will function throughout life. The embryo will respond to prodding, although it has no consciousness at this stage of development. The brain's higher functions do not develop until much later in pregnancy.

10 weeks: The embryo is now called a fetus. Its face looks human; its gender may be detectable via ultrasound.

13 weeks or 3 months: The fetus is about 3 inches long and weighs about an ounce. Fingernails and bones can be seen. Over 90 per cent of all abortions are performed before this stage.

17 weeks or 3.9 months: It is 8" long and weighs about a half pound. The fetus' movements may begin to be felt. Its heartbeat can usually be detected.

22 weeks or 5 months: 12" long and weighing about a pound, the fetus has hair on its head. Its movements can be felt. An abortion is usually unavailable at this gestational age because of state and province medical society regulations, except under very unusual circumstances. Half-way through the 22nd week, the fetus' lungs may be developed to the point where it would have a miniscule chance to live on its own. State laws and medical association regulations generally outlaw almost all abortions beyond 20 or 21 weeks gestation. *"A baby born during the 22nd week has a 14.8 per cent chance of survival. And about half of these survivors are brain-damaged, either by lack of oxygen (from poor initial respiration) or too much oxygen (from the ventilator). Neonatologists predict that no baby will ever be viable before the 22nd week, because before then the lungs are not fully formed."*

Of course, if someone develops an artificial womb, then this limit could change suddenly.

Fetal survival rate: "*Most babies at 22 weeks are not resuscitated because survival without major disability is so rare. A baby's chances for survival increases 3-4 per cent per day between 23 and 24 weeks of gestation and about 2-3 per cent per day between 24 and 26 weeks of gestation. After 26 weeks the rate of survival increases at a much slower rate because survival is high already.*"

26 weeks or 6 months: The fetus 14" long and almost two pounds. The lungs' bronchioles develop. Interlinking of the brain's neurons begins. The higher functions of the fetal brain turn on for the first time. Some rudimentary brain waves can be detected. The fetus will be able to feel pain for the first time. It has become conscious of its surroundings. The fetus has become a sentient human life for the first time.

7 months: 16" long and weighing about three pounds. Regular brain waves are detectable which are similar to those in adults.

8 months: 18" long and weighing about 5 pounds.

9 months: 20" long and with an average weight of 7 pounds, a full-term fetus is typically born about this time.

DELIVERY PROCESS

Embryonic Period

The embryonic time comprises 56 days, i.e., 8 weeks from the moment of fertilisation. This time span is divided into 23 Carnegie stages and the stage classification is based solely on morphologic features. Carnegie stages are thus neither directly dependent on the chronological age nor on the size of the embryo. This can be illustrated by two examples: The closure of the rostral neuropore occurs by definition in stage 11 and that of the caudal neuropore in stage 12. Further, between the 25th and 32nd days of the pregnancy, the stages are determined according to the number of the somites <9-13> that have been engendered. The individual stages thus differ in how long they last.

During the embryonic period most of the organ systems are established and this with an enormous rapidity. Cell divisions, movement and differentiation are the basic processes taking place during this phase. It is thus hardly surprising that this pregnancy phase is very vulnerable and that deformities are produced most often during this time. The type of deformity depends on the embryonic developmental stage.

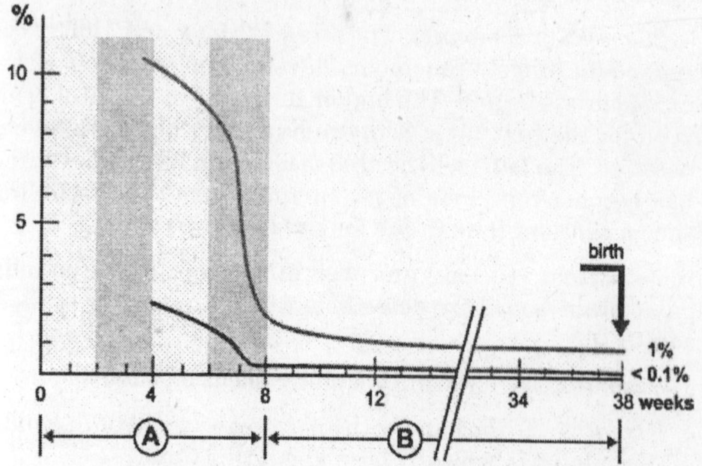

Fig. 3.1: Incidence of deformities during pregnancy

Fig. 3.1 Segment A represents the embryonic period in which the embryo is especially sensitive with respect to deformities. Within the first eight weeks, the incidence of deformities (blue curve), that lead to miscarriages, decreases from more than 10 per cent to 1 per cent during the fetal period (B). The frequency of neural tube defects decreases from 2.5 per cent to 0.1 per cent (green curve) by the end of the embryonic period.

Fetal Period

According to estimates, over 90 per cent of the 4500 designated structures of the adult body are already established—and can be distinguished—during the embryonic period. During the fetal period the organs that formed during the embryonic period grow and differentiate (organogenesis).

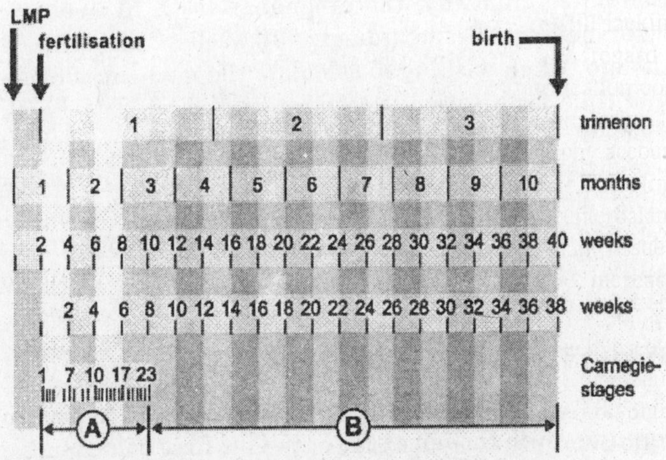

Fig. 3.2: Time calculations during pregnancy

Fig. 3.2 The schematic diagram shows the various time periods during the entire pregnancy. LMP = Last Menstruation Period. The embryonic period (A) lasts 8 weeks and the fetal period (B) from the 9th week to the birth, i.e., 30 weeks.

Figure 3.2 shows the various temporal phases during a pregnancy. A rough classification is made by assigning trimesters (trimenon). The LMP (Last Menstruation Period) is not the real beginning of the pregnancy but serves as a point of reference for determining the date of ovulation and thus the moment of fertilisation. Normally this occurs 14 days after the beginning of menstruation, but can vary a lot temporally. From the time of the last period, one estimates 40 weeks after the last menstruation in order to determine the approximate date of birth (the second and third grid marks represent the lunar month [of 28 days] or 4 weeks). On average, though, the duration of an actual pregnancy amounts to 266 days or 38 weeks (fourth grid). The embryonic period (A) lasts 8 weeks and the fetal period (B) from the 9th week to the birth.

In obstetrics the pregnancy weeks (PW) are normally reckoned from the date of the Last Menstrual Period (LMP).

This is a point in time that many women can easily remember. Computed this way, the pregnancy lasts 40 weeks and the embryonic period—accordingly—10 weeks. Caution is advisable, though, when wishing to calculate the moment of ovulation—and thus fertilisation, closely connected with it—because the moment of ovulation can vary and depends on many factors (conditioned by the environment and psychological aspects). In embryology the temporal indices (i.e., the PW), therefore, always refer to the moment of fertilisation even though in practical midwifery the time following the LMP is still used for computations.

Fetus at 8 Weeks

After the 8th week, the fetus takes on typical human features, even though at the end of the first trimenon, the head is still relatively large in appearance. The eyes shift to the front and the ears and nasal saddle are formed. The eyelids are also clearly recognisable now. On the body, fine lanugo hairs are formed, which at the time of birth are replaced by terminal hairs. The physiologic umbilical hernia that arises in the embryonic period <15-20> has mostly disappeared. In the second trimenon the mother feels the first movements of the child. In the last trimenon the subcutaneous fatty tissue is formed and stretches the still wrinkled skin of the fetus. The skin becomes covered more and more with vernix caseosa. This is a whitish, greasy substance and consists of flaked off epithelial cells and sebaceous gland secretions. In neonatology this vernix caseosa is an important criterion for judging the maturity of the child. If the birth occurs post-term, it disappears again.

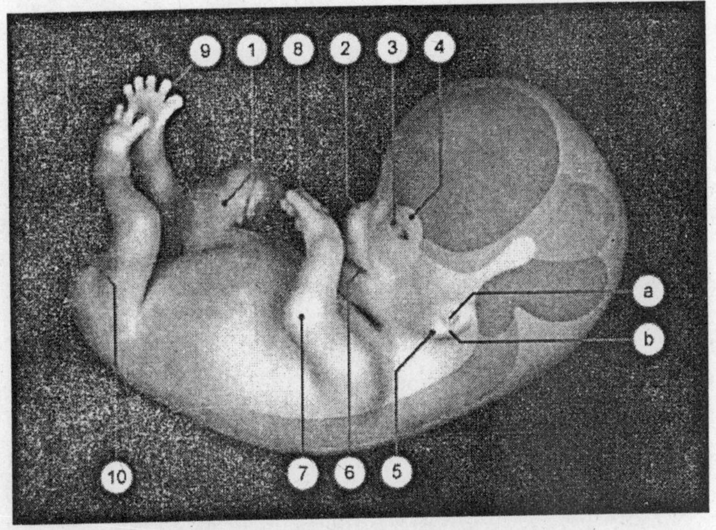

Fig. 3.3: The fetus still has a large head in relation to the rest of the body

1. Umbilcal cord with hernia
2. Nose
3. Eye
4. Eyelid
5. Ear (a: tragus, b: antitragus)
6. Mouth
7. Elbow
8. Finger
9. Toes
10. Atrophied embryonic tail bud

Childbirth (also called labour, birth, *partus* or parturition) is the culmination of a human pregnancy or gestation period with the delivery of one or more newborn infants from a woman's uterus. The process of human childbirth is categorised in 3 stages of labour. The first stage accomplishes the shortening and then the dilation of the cervix. It is deemed to have started when the cervix is 3 cm dilated, and ends with full dilation. Contractions begin in the first stage of labour although they may be irregular and sporadic at first. The second stage, often called the pushing stage, starts when the cervix is fully dilated and ends with the expulsion of the fetus. In the third stage, the placenta detaches from the uterine wall and is expelled through the birth canal. Preceding the onset of labour is a period called the latent phase. This phase may last many days, and the contractions are an intensification of the Braxton Hicks contractions that start around 26 weeks gestation. Latent phase ends with the onset of active first stage labour.

The Mechanics of Birth

Because humans are bipedal with an erect stance and humans have relatively the biggest head and shoulders to the size of the pelvis of any species, humans fetuses are adapted to make birth possible.

The erect posture causes the weight of the abdominal contents to thrust on the pelvic floor, a complex structure which must not only support this weight but allow three channels to pass through it: the urethra, the vagina and the rectum. The relatively large head and shoulders require a specific sequence of manoeuvres to occur for the bony head and shoulders to pass through the bony ring of the pelvis. If these manoeuvres fail, the progress of labour is arrested. All changes in the soft tissues of the cervix and the birth canal are entirely dependent on the successful completion of these six manoeuvers:

- Engagement of the fetal head in the transverse position. The baby is looking across the pelvis at one or other of the mother's hips;
- Descent and flexion of the fetal head;
- Internal rotation. The fetal head rotates 90 degrees to the occipito-anterior so that the baby's face is towards the mother's rectum;

- Delivery by extension. The fetal head passes out of the birth canal. Its head is tilted backwards so that its forehead leads the way through the vagina;
- Restitution. The fetal head turns through 45 degrees to restore its normal relationship with the shoulders, which are still at an angle;
- External rotation. The shoulders repeat the corkscrew movements of the head, which can be seen in the final movements of the fetal head.

These movements are all due to the relationship of the bony head and shoulders of the fetus to the bony ring of the mother's pelvis and are independent of any changes in the maternal soft tissues.

The latent phase of labour causes confusion with many. Latent phase may last many days and the contractions are an intensification of the Braxton-Hicks contractions that start around 26 weeks gestation. Cervical effacement occurs during the closing weeks of pregnancy and is usually complete or near complete, by the end of latent phase. Cervical effacement is the incorporation of the cervix to form the lower segment of the uterus. The muscular portion of the uterus is the upper segment, and is made of non-striated muscle. The lower segment of the uterus has no muscles and is comprised of the cervix itself, which becomes massively stretched and thinned out. This cervical effacement will usually be accomplished fully prior to the onset of labour. The degree of cervical effacement may be felt during a vaginal examination. A 'long' cervix implies that not much has been taken into the lower segment, and vice versa for a 'short' cervix. Latent phase ends with the onset of active first stage; when the cervix is about 3 cm dilated.

First Stage: Contractions

The first stage of labour is an active stage and should not be confused with the latent phase of labour. The first stage of labour starts classically when the effaced cervix is 3 cm dilated. There is variation in this point as some patients may present a little before this point with active contraction, or later, without regular contractions. The onset of actual labour is defined when the cervix begins to progressively dilate. Rupture of the membranes, or a blood stained 'show' may or may not occur at around this stage.

Uterine muscles form opposing spirals from the top of the upper segment of the uterus to its junction with the lower segment. During effacement, the cervix becomes incorporated into the lower segment. During a contraction, these muscles contract causing shortening of the upper segment and drawing upwards of the lower segment, in a gradual expulsive motion. This draws the cervix up over the baby's head. Full dilatation is reached when the cervix is the size of the baby's head; at around 10 cm dilation for a term baby.

The duration of labour varies widely, but active phase averages some 8 hours for women giving birth to their first child ("primiparae") and 4 hours for women who have already given birth ("multiparae").

Second Stage: Delivery

This stage begins when the cervix is fully dilated, and ends when the baby is finally delivered. At the beginning of the normal second stage, the head is fully engaged in the pelvis; the widest diameter of the head has successfully passed through the pelvic brim. Ideally it has successfully also passed below the interspinous diameter. This is the narrowest part of the pelvis. If these have been accomplished, all that will remain is for the fetal head to pass below the pubic arch and out through the introituses. This is assisted by the additional maternal efforts of "bearing down". The fetal head is seen to 'crown' as the labia part. At this point the woman may feel a burning or stinging sensation.

Delivery of the fetal head signals the successful completion of the fourth mechanism of labour (delivery by extension), and is followed by the fifth and sixth mechanisms (restitution and external rotation). The second stage of labour will vary to some extent, depending on how successfully the preceding tasks have been accomplished.

Abnormalities of Second Stage

Delays in second stage may be caused by:

- Mal-presentation of the fetal head;
- Failure of descent of the fetal head through the pelvic brim or the interspinous diameter;
- Poor uterine contraction strength;
- A big baby and a small pelvis;
- Shoulder dystocia.

These factors will lead to prolongation of the second stage of labour. Secondary changes may be observed: swelling of the tissues, maternal exhaustion, fetal heart rate abnormalities. Left untreated, severe complications include death of mother or baby, and genito-vaginal fistula. These are commonly seen in Third World countries where births are often unattended or attended by poorly trained community members.

Third Stage: Placenta

In this stage, the uterus expels the placenta (afterbirth). Maternal blood loss is limited by the compression of the spiral arteries of the uterus as they pass though the lattice-like uterine muscles of the upper segment. Normal blood loss is less than 600 ml. The placenta is usually delivered within 15 minutes of the baby being born.

Management of Third Stage

The third stage can be managed either expectantly or actively. Active management utilises oxytocic agents to augment uterine muscular contraction. This contraction acts both to shear off the placental attachment and to compress the spiral arteries. Controlled cord traction assists with rapid delivery of the placenta. Expectant management allows the placenta to be expelled without assistance.

After the Birth

Medical professionals typically recommend breastfeeding of the first milk, colostrum, to reduce postpartum bleeding/

haemorrhage in the mother, and to pass immunities and other benefits to the baby. Many cultures feature initiation rites for newborns, such as naming ceremonies, baptism, and others.

Mothers are often allowed a period where they are relieved of their normal duties to recover from childbirth. The length of this period varies. In China it is 30 days and is referred to as "doing the month" or "sitting month" (see Postpartum period). In some other countries, taking time off from work to care for a newborn is called "maternity leave" and can vary from a few days to several months.

When the amniotic sac has not ruptured during labour or pushing, the infant can be born with the membranes intact. This is referred to as "being born in the caul." The caul is harmless and its membranes are easily broken and wiped away. In medieval times, and in some cultures still today, a caul was seen as a sign of good fortune for the baby, even giving the child psychic gifts such as clairvoyance, and in some cultures was seen as protection against drowning. The caul was often impressed onto paper and stored away as an heirloom for the child. With the advent of modern obstetrics, premature artificial rupture of the membranes has become common, so babies are rarely born in the caul.

Orgasm during Childbirth

Some women experience orgasm during childbirth. There are similarities between the process of orgasm and childbirth; both involve involuntary contractions of some of the same muscles. Orgasm releases endorphins which can mediate the pain of labour, as well as the hormone oxytocin, which is known to play an important role in labour as well as mother-child attachment. Some people have speculated that sexual repression, in particular, the repression of women's sexuality, may be holding more women back both from having an orgasmic experience with childbirth, and from accepting and sharing the experience when they do have it. One doctor commented that he had seen a few women have an orgasmic experience during birth, but speculated that many women may interpret them as pain because they are so conditioned to expect pain.

Pain

Pain levels reported by women in labour vary widely. This variation is not dissimilar for perceived pain in other situations. Pain levels seem to be influenced by fear and anxiety levels, experience with prior childbirth, cultural ideas of childbirth and pain, mobility during labour and the support given during labour.

Non-medical Pain Control

Some women prefer to avoid analgesic medication during childbirth. They still can try to alleviate labour pain using psychological preparation, education, massage, hypnosis, or water therapy in a tub or shower. Some women like to have someone to support them during labour and birth, such as the father of the baby, the woman's mother, a sister, a close friend or a partner. Some women deliver in a squatting or crawling position in order to more effectively push during the second stage and so that gravity can aid the descent of the baby through the birth canal.

The human body also has a chemical response to pain, by releasing endorphins. Endorphins are present before, during, and immediately after childbirth. Some homebirth advocates believe that this hormone can induce feelings of pleasure and euphoria during childbirth, reducing the risk of maternal depression some weeks later. Water birth is an option chosen by some women for pain relief during labour and childbirth, and some studies have shown water-birth in an uncomplicated pregnancy to reduce the need for analgesia, without evidence of increased risk to mother or newborn. Hot water tubs are available in many hospitals and birthing centers.

Meditation and mind medicine techniques for the use of pain control during labour and delivery. These techniques are used in conjunction with progressive muscle relaxation and many other forms of relaxation for the mind and body to aid in pain control for women during childbirth. One such technique is the use of hypnosis in childbirth.

Medical Pain Control

Different measures for pain control have varying degrees of success and side effects to the woman and her baby. In some countries of Europe, doctors commonly prescribe inhaled nitrous oxide gas for pain control; in the UK, midwives may use this gas without a doctor's prescription. Pethidine (with or without promethazine) may be used early in labour, as well as other opioids, but if given too close to birth there is a risk of respiratory depression in the infant.

Popular medical pain control in hospitals includes the regional anaesthetics epidural blocks, and spinal anaesthesia. Epidural analgesia is a safe and effective method of relieving pain in labour, but is associated with longer labour, more operative intervention (particularly instrument delivery), and increases in cost. Medicine administered via epidural can cross the placenta and enter the bloodstream of the fetus. Epidural analgesia has no statistically significant impact on the risk of caesarean section, and does not appear to have an immediate effect on neonatal status as determined by Apgar scores.

COMPLICATIONS AND RISKS

(A) Complications and Risks of Birth

Complications can occur during childbirth. Infant deaths (*neonatal deaths* from birth to 28 days, or *perinatal deaths* if including fetal deaths at 28 weeks gestation and later) are around 1 per cent in modernised countries. The maternal mortality (MMR) rate varies from 9/100,000 live births in the US and Europe, to 900/100,000 live births in Sub-Saharan Africa. The "natural" mortality rate of childbirth—where nothing is done to avert maternal death—has been estimated as being between 1,000 and 1,500 deaths per 100,000 births.

The most important factors affecting mortality in childbirth are adequate nutrition and access to quality medical care ("access" is affected both by the cost of available care, and distance from health services). "Medical care" in this context does not refer specifically to treatment in hospitals, but simply routine prenatal care and the presence, at the birth, of an attendant with birthing skills.

A 1983-1989 study by the Texas Department of Health highlighted the differences in neonatal mortality (NMR) between high risk and low risk pregnancies. NMR was 0.57 per cent for doctor-attended high risk births, and 0.19 per cent for low risk births attended by non-nurse midwives. Conversely, some studies demonstrate a higher peri-natal mortality rate with assisted home births. Around 80 per cent of pregnancies are low-risk. Factors that may make a birth high risk include pre-maturity, high blood pressure, gestational diabetes and a previous cesarean section.

Birthing complication may be maternal or fetal, and long term or short term.

Maternal Risks

Haemorrhage is still the biggest killer of birthing mothers in the world today especially in the developing world. Heavy blood loss leads to hypovolemic shock, insufficient perfusion of vital organs and death if not rapidly treated. Blood transfusion may be life saving.

Infection remains a major cause of mortality and morbidity in the developing world today.

Vaginal birth injury with visible tears or episiotomies is common. Internal tissue tearing as well as nerve damage to the pelvic structures lead in a proportion of women to problems with pro-lapse, incontinence of stool or urine and sexual dysfunction. Fifteen per cent of women become incontinent, to some degree, of stool or urine after normal delivery, this number rising considerably after these women reach menopause.

Vaginal birth injury is a necessary, but not sufficient, cause of all non hysterectomy related pro-lapse in later life. Risk factors for significant vaginal birth injury include: a baby weighing more than nine pounds the use of forceps or vacuum for delivery. These markers are more likely to be signals for other abnormalities as forceps or vacuum are not used in normal deliveries. Hormones and enzymes work together to produce ligamentous relaxation and widening of the symphysis pubis during the last trimester of pregnancy. Most girdle pain occurs before birthing, and is know as diastasis of the pubic symphysis. Predisposing factors for girdle pain include maternal obesity.

(B) Fetal Complications

Intrapartum asphyxia: The term *Fetal distress* is emotive and misleading. True intrapartum asphyxia is the impairment of oxygen to the brain and vital tissues during the progress of labour. This may exist in a pregnancy already impaired by maternal or fetal disease, or may rarely arise *de novo* in labour. True intrapartum asphyxia is not as common as previously believed, and is usually accompanied by multiple other symptoms during the immediate period after delivery. Monitoring might show up problems during birthing, but the interpretation and use of monitoring devices is complex and prone to misinterpretation.

Mechanical Fetal Injury

Risk factors for fetal birth injury include fetal macrosomia (big baby), maternal obesity, the need for instrumental delivery, and an inexperienced attendant. Specific situations that can contribute to birth injury include breech presentation and shoulder dystocia. Most fetal birth injuries resolve without long term harm, but brachial plexus injury may lead to Erb's palsy.

Neonatal Infection

Neonates are prone to infection in the first month of life. Some organisms such as S. agalactiae (Group B Streptococcus) or (GBS) are more prone to cause these occasionally fatal infections. Risk factors for GBS infection include:

Twins and Multiple Births

Twins can be delivered vaginally. In some cases twin delivery is done in a larger delivery room or in theatre, just in case complications occur e.g. both twins born vaginally—one comes normally but the other is breech and/or helped by a forceps/ventouse delivery. One twin born could be born vaginally and the other could be by caesarean section. If the twins are joined at any part of the body—called conjoined twins, delivery is mostly by caesarean section.

Professionals Associated with Childbirth

Doulas are assistants who support mothers during pregnancy, labour, birth, and postpartum. They are not medical attendants; rather, they provide emotional support and non-medical pain relief for women during labour.

Maternal-fetal medicine specialists are experts in managing and treating high-risk pregnancy and delivery. They are usually also obstetricians.

Midwives provide care to low-risk pregnant mothers. Midwives may be licenced and registered, or may be lay practitioners. Jurisdictions with legislated midwives will typically have a registering and disciplinary body, such as a College of Midwifery.

Registered midwives are trained to assist a mother with labour and birth, either through direct-entry or nurse-midwifery programmes. Lay midwives, who are usually not licenced or registered, typically gain experience through apprenticeship with other lay midwives.

Obstetricians provide care for normal and abnormal births and pathological labour conditions. Obstetricians are trained surgeons, so they can undertake surgical procedures relating to childbirth. Such procedures include cesarean sections, episiotomies, or assisted delivery. Most obstetricians also provide gynaecological care, and may have a primary, well-woman, care element to their practices.

Obstetric nurses assist midwives, doctors, women, and babies prior to, during, and after the birth process, in the hospital system. Some midwives are also obstetric nurses. Obstetric nurses hold various certifications and typically undergo additional obstetric training in addition to standard nursing training.

Socio-cultural Aspects

In most cultures, childbirth is considered to be the beginning of a person's life, and their age is defined relative to it. Some families view the placenta as a special part of birth, since it has been the child's life support for so many months. Some parents like to see and touch this organ. In some cultures, parents plant a tree along with the placenta on the child's first birthday. The placenta may be eaten by the newborn's family, ceremonially or otherwise. The exact location in which childbirth takes place is an important factor in determining nationality, in particular for birth aboard aircraft and ships.

Psychological Aspects

Childbirth can be a stressful event. As with any stressful event, strong emotions can be brought to the surface. Some women report symptoms compatible with post-traumatic stress disorder (PTSD) after birth. Between 70 and 80 per cent of mothers in the United States report some feelings of sadness or "baby blues" after childbirth. Postpartum depression may develop in some women; about 10 per cent of mothers in the United States are diagnosed with this condition. Abnormal and persistent fear of childbirth is known as tokophobia. Preventative group therapy has proven effective as a prophylactic treatment for postpartum depression.

There are some who argue that childbirth is stressful for the infant. Stresses associated with breech birth, such as asphyxiation, may affect the infant's brain.

Partner and Other Support

There is increasing evidence to show that the participation of the woman's partner in the birth leads to better birth and also post-birth outcomes, providing the partner does not exhibit excessive anxiety. Research also shows that when a woman in labour was supported by a female helper such as a family member or doula during labour, she had less need for chemical pain relief, the likelihood of caesarean section was reduced, use of forceps and other instrumental deliveries were reduced and there was a reduction in the length of labour and the baby had a higher Apgar score.

It is the traditional history of home labour that makes The Netherlands an attractive site for studies related to birth. One third of all baby deliveries there are still happening at home in contrast with other western industrialised countries.

Apparently, Dutch fathers have been in the scene of labour for a long time as can be observed in paintings from the 17th and 18th centuries. It was found that fathers can have different roles during birth and that little is said about the conflicts between partners or partners and professionals. Among other findings were also: the interpretation of the presence of fathers during birth as a modern version of the anthropological couvade ritual to ease the woman's pain; the majority of fathers did not perceive any limitation to participate in their childbirth and upper generations did not play an important rule in the transmission of knowledge about birth to those fathers but the wives, feminine acquaintances and midwives.

Postnatal (Latin for 'after birth', from *post* meaning "after" and *natalis* meaning "of birth") is the period beginning immediately after the birth of a child and extending for about six weeks. The period is also known as postpartum period and, less commonly, puerperium.

Biologically, it is the time after birth, a time in which the mother's body, including hormone levels and uterus size, return to pre-pregnancy conditions. Lochia is post-partum vaginal discharge, containing blood, mucus, and placental tissue.

During the first stages of this period, the newborn also starts his/her adaptation to extra-uterine life, the most significant physiological transition until death. In scientific literature the term is commonly abbreviated to PX. So that 'day P5' should be read as 'the fifth day after birth'.

(C) The Postnatal Complications

A woman in the Western world who is delivering in a hospital may leave the hospital as soon as she is medically stable and chooses to leave, which can be as early as a few hours postpartum, though the average for spontaneous vaginal delivery (SVD) is 1-2 days, and the average caesarean section postnatal stay is 3-4 days. During this time bleeding, bowel and bladder function, and baby care are monitored.

Physical Aspects

The mother is assessed for tears, and is sutured if necessary. Also, she may suffer from constipation or haemorrhoids, both of which would be managed. The bladder is also assessed for infection, retention and any problems in the muscles. The major focus of postpartum care is ensuring that the woman is healthy and capable of taking care of her newborn, equipped with all the information she needs about breastfeeding, reproductive health and contraception, and the imminent life adjustment.

Some medical conditions may occur post-natally, such as Sheehan Syndrome. In some cases, this adjustment is not made easily, and hormonal disturbances may lead to postnatal depression or even puerperal psychosis.

Psychological Aspects

Postnatal depression ("Baby blues") is very common, with approximately 50 per cent of women suffering from it, potentially as early as 24 hours postpartum. It is usually limited in duration, lasting 36 to 48 hours. Apart from empathy and support from caregivers and family, treatment is not required. Approximately 10-20 per cent of women will suffer the symptoms of major depression, and should be treated accordingly. Postpartum depression may be the response to the hormonal changes and life adjustment the woman goes through immediately after childbirth.

Postnatal Psychosis (also known as puerperal psychosis), is a more severe form of mental illness than postpartum depression.

Care provided by a postpartum doula supports the mother, assists with breastfeeding and baby care which enhances her confidence, helping to lessen her chances of developing postpartum depression or other postpartum mood disorders.

In some East Asian cultures, such as Chinese and Vietnamese, there is a traditional custom of postpartum confinement known in English as doing the month or sitting the month. Confinement traditionally lasts 30 days, although regional variants may last 40, 60 or as many as 100 days. This tradition combines prescribed foods with a number of restrictions on activities considered to be harmful to the woman's recovering body. Family elders or (more recently) health professionals help the woman to recover after parturition.

Prohibited activities include washing one's hair, bathing, climbing steps, touching cold water, reading, and crying; sexual activity is prohibited, and the woman is not supposed be exposed to the wind or to sew. She is not supposed to consume anything cold, anything hard, any salt, any plain water, or anything containing alcohol or other foods considered to have strong medicinal properties.

SECTION TWO

BODY IMAGE—TRIBAL PERCEPTIONS

In his book captioned, "The Thakars of Sahyadri" Chaphekar L.N. (1961: 79) illustrated the ideas of the tribals regarding the physical world from an emic perspective. He presented the analogy of Thakar rationale comparing human bodies with plants.

- According to Thakars, plants like human beings have emotions. They experience joy and sorrow. If a plant is struck with an axe it shrieks.
- Life of a plant is in roots. The roots give the tree strength and support.
- Plants also need water, air and light.
- There are males and female plants.
- Male plants yield bigger fruits than female plants.
- The Thakar describes the human body in one of his riddles as the tree with branches below and truck above. The human system is believed to function in a way similar to the working of the animal system; the human bodily system contains the same parts as the body of a vertebrate animal. Except for the obvious differences, the description of the human body is the same as that of animal system. (Chaphekar L.N. 1961:6).

From the view point of the Thakars as reported by L.N.Chaphekar the concept sounds logical, because they do not aware of what a skeletal system is? Whatever they know human body is according to what they observe among animals they hunt and plants they see. The point which the authors here are trying to bring to the notice of readers is that there is a difference between the knowledge of a tribal regarding body image and human reproduction system, from that of an educated person.

Furthermore, Tribhuwan Robin (1998) in his book 'Medical world of Tribals' revealed how Thakars associate human body as a natural, social, cosmic and spiritual symbol in various healing ritual contexts. Well, that's how the tribals view or understand human body. Chapter Four of this book throws light on this aspect.

PERCEPTIONS AND IDEAS ABOUT THE PROCESS OF CONCEPTION

Tribhuwan's study (1998) reveals the process of conception among the Thakars. According to them a woman's egg is equated with a flower, which is released by her during the sexual intercourse. This flower is fertilised by a speck of (spermatozoid) and released by a man during the intercourse. The fertilised flower, then grows as foetus in the woman's womb.

Interestingly the speck of sperm and the flower (egg) for both males and the females is stored in two worms that are situated right beneath the fronto-nasal suture in the forehead. These worms release flower in case of a female and speck (spermatozoid) in case of males. They run down from the head and come out of the penis and vagina respectively. The fertilised flower than grows in the womb.

Role of Hormones in Reproduction System

Unlike the scientific world that understands the role of hormones in reproduction, tribals do not know what hormones are? Neither do they understand their role in human reproduction system. Tribhuwan's study (1998) however revealed the role of water, air, light and heat in the body in mobilising and accelerating the process of human reproduction.

Stages of Growth

A Thakar midwife and a woman know that the full period of pregnancy is nine months and nine days. They are also aware that some children are born premature. Tribal concept of fertilisation and formation of embryo are drawn from observations of pregnant women. The TBAs are aware of the stages of growth and development of foetus. They calculate the stages of growth on the basis of lunar calendar. When a girl shows signs of vomiting nausea etc. the calculations of embryonic formations and growth of foetus by TBAs begins. Some of the elderly women in the family too are expert in this area.

Delivery Process

When a woman feels that she is near her time, she goes home, changes her sari, wraps a piece of cloth round her loins, and lies down supine on a *ghongadi* or rough blanket in the inner chamber, resting her head on a folded cloth. There are no previous preparations. Instances of women delivered outside the house are exceptional.

Messengers are then sent to fetch the local midwife and her assistant who is called a *potdhari* – one who holds the belly. They are both Thakar women. A midwife is paid about a rupee for her services and a *potdhari* about half as much. The knowledge they have gained is all through experience. A *potdhari* is an apprentice who expects to become a midwife in due course.

The mother continues to lie supine till she is delivered of her child. Charpoys are not used till the woman has delivered. The ghongadi at this time is moved up, the bare hypo gastric and public region resting on the floor. The midwife squats at the woman's feet and the potdhari by her side. The potdhari massages her belly downwards and the midwife is ready to guide the emerging child. The parturient woman holds her breath and makes an effort to relieve herself. At the same time the potdhari gently massages downwards and the midwife pulls out the infant.

On the presentation of the child, the midwife, if necessary, gently pulls the umbilical cord to bring out the placenta. She cuts the cord with a sickle and ties it with a piece of white unused string. The sickle is then placed at the head of the child and under the hammock in which the child is placed on the fifth day. A cubit-deep hole is dug just outside the house on the other side of the place, where the mother and child are to be bathed, and the after birth is buried there. The afterbirth is placed on a *palas* leaf and some rice is put over it. It is then placed in the ditch by the midwife. The ditch is usually dug by a woman. After filling up the ditch the midwife places heavy stones over it as a safeguard against dog.

If there is much delay, or the delivery is difficult, charmed ash is brought from a *bhagat* and applied to the forehead of the parturient woman. Another measure is to wet a part of her husband's loin-cloth in a little water and to give the water to the ailing woman to drink. Placing herbs under the woman's head is also supposed to be efficacious.

After delivery the woman sits with her legs folded, pressing the vagina with her right heel to prevent prolapsed of the uterus. In the case of a prolapsed uterus the woman is laid down and the uterus is pushed in. The woman is then seated on a hot brick covered with a piece of cloth.

After depositing the afterbirth the midwife bathes the mother and the child with hot water. Prior to her bath, the mother is made to stand, arms up, and the midwife massages her belly with the right knee to force out blood. The bath over, the midwife changes the loin-cloth of the mother, this time using a bigger piece of cloth which is worn tighter and is well tucked in. The mother then warms herself at the fire and, while warming herself, she chews some *ova* and copra and blows the vapour on the navel and head of the child. She then eats the *ova* and copra and drinks a little hot water. When she feels sufficiently warm, she is fed some gruel of rice or *vari*, and is then allowed to rest.

The bath, the feed and the rest make her feel fresh and comfortable enough to feed the child. If the child is asleep when the mother is ready to give in its first feed, it is awakened. This is necessary, as otherwise it is thought the child will not learn to suck. The usual position for the first feed is for the mother to sit down and hold the child in her lap. *Dudhakand* or milk-tuber, available in the jungle, is supposed to be efficacious in increasing the supply of milk. It is given to both women and to dairy-animals.

For five days after child birth the mother is fed only rice or vari gruel. She must eat a moderate quantity of it. She cannot eat salt and must keep indoors during this period. After five days she is given rice, pulse and milk. For two or three weeks, according to her health, her diet excludes all excesses and is strictly vegetarian. It is only afterwards that she is given, if means allow, flesh of fowl, eggs or milk to help her recuperate.

No period of impurity after giving birth is observed by members of the family. They restrict their activities to household work, however, and refrain especially from setting fire to *rab* ground burnt for sowing, from carrying a dead body and from offering *dhan* in obsequies. This restriction continues for five days.

Knowledge About Complications and Risks

Complications and risks in child birth are managed only by highly skilled and experienced TBAs. With the expansion of PHCs and private hospitals at the tahsil level, tribal TBAs who are not too experienced advice the woman's relatives to take her to the PHC/hospital. However, many women prefer to deliver children in their houses.

A survey conducted by T.R.and T.I. Pune (2000:28) in Nandurbar district revealed that 93.31 per cent of the deliveries among tribal families studied were conducted at home. Table given below reveals it all.

Table 3.1

Place of Delivery

Sr. No.	*Place of Delivery*	*Number*	*Percentage*
1.	At home	142	99.31%
2.	Did not respond	1	0.69%
	Total	**143**	**100**

The reasons given by respondents as to why deliveries conducted at home are:

(i) The umbilical cord has to be buried next to the house. Burial of umbilical cord symbolizes the attachment of child to the house and family;

(ii) On the fifth day after the birth of a child the midwife, performs the ceremony of worshipping the mother goddess. The ritual is performed at home;

(iii) A few women (educated) said that hospital expenses were too high.

95 per cent and 3.52 per cent of the deliveries were conducted by traditional female (Huvarki) and male birth attendants, in the house of the tribals. This is because the TBA attends birth rituals. Secondly, according to the tribal women TBAs are more accessible, arrive in time, are available at all times of the right and also they are preferable to the paramedical staff.

Table 3.2

Personnel who conduct Delivery

Sr. No.	*Birth Attendants*	*Number*	*Percentage*
1.	Female Traditional Birth Attendant	136	95.0%
2.	Male T.B.A.	5	3.52%
3.	A.N.M.	1	0.69%
4.	Did not Respond	1	0.69%
	Total	**143**	**100%**

Studies by following authors also reveal that the percentage of deliveries at home in tribal societies is very high.

- A report by Tribal Research and Training Institute (2000:18) captioned "Dying children" reported that 96 per cent of deliveries in selected tribal families were at home while 4 per cent in P.H.C./Sub Centre. The same study revealed that 92 per cent of the deliveries were attended by TBAs.
- In his study, captioned "Medical World by Tribals", Tribhuwan Robin (1998) revealed that over 90 per cent of the deliveries among the Thakars of Karjat were conducted at home and 92 per cent of them conducted by TBAs.
- A survey captioned, "Socio-economic Status and Development Needs of the Katkaris: A Case Study, by Tribhuwan Robin (2006) states that deliveries of all the 14 families studied were conducted at home by the midwife.
- Y.P.S. Tomar and Tribhuwan Robin (2005:52) in their book entitled "The Mavchis of Nandurbar: A lesser known Tribe, revealed the 71 per cent of the deliveries among the Mavchis were conducted at home and 89.62 per cent of them were handled by TBAs.

Age at Marriage

Studies by Jain N.S. and Tribhuwan Robin (1995, 1996), Tribhuwan Robin 1998; Bhanu B.V. and Kulkarni L.V. (1995) revealed that the average age at marriage for girls among tribals is from 14 to 17 and for boys it is from 15 to 20, with few exceptions. An undernourished girl gets married at an early age and produces a low birth weight child. She faces problems during delivery.

Illiteracy among Tribal Women

The table given below clearly indicates that the literacy rate among tribal females is very low as compared to females of general population. In fact, it is pertinent to note that there is a big gap of literacy rate among tribal and non-tribal women. It is widening decade after decade. No wonder why tribal women face gynecological problems.

Table 3.3

General & Tribal Literacy Rates in Maharashtra during five decades

Sr. No	*Year*	*General*			*Tribal*		
		Male	*Female*	*Total*	*Male*	*Female*	*Total*
1.	1961	42.04	16.76	29.82	12.55	1.75	7.21
2.	1971	51.04	26.43	39.13	19.06	4.21	11.74
3.	1981	58.65	34.67	47.02	32.38	11.94	22.29
4.	1991	76.56	52.30	49.08	49.08	24.08	36.77
5.	2001	86.60	67.00	76.90	67.00	43.10	52.20

BPL Status

The Tribal Research and Training Institute, Pune conducted a Bench Mark Survey in 1981 that revealed 94 per cent of the tribals in Maharashtra were below the poverty line. The same institute conducted Bench Mark Survey in 2001 which revealed that 92 per cent of tribals in the State were below the poverty line. This means that during a span of 16 years only 2 per cent made the difference. Table Number 3.4 depicts I.T.D.P. wise tribal Below Poverty Line families in Maharashtra.

Food Scarcity

Majority of tribals are small scale cultivators. They cultivate for six months and work as agricultural labourers or daily wage labourers for the remaining six months. Production for consumption and not distribution is one of the salient features of their economic organisation. Studies have revealed that food grains produced by them are enough for 4 to 6 months.

Tribal Research and Training Institute, Pune conducted a study in (2002: 10). The table below indicates the number of month's food availability from their own land. Out of the 143 families, 123 (86%) were food deficit. As many as 78 per cent of the households had a food deficit of 6 months or more. This was the food deficit from their own farms.

Table 3.4

I.T.D.P. wise Below Poverty Line tribal families in Maharashtra

Sr. No.	*I.T.D.P.*	*S.T. Families*		*Percentage of families below poverty line (figures in Col.4 to Col.No.3)*
		Total	*Below poverty line*	
1.	Thane (Dahanu)	66447	59595	89.69
2.	Thane (Jawhar)	46556	40939	87.93
3.	Thane (Shahapur)	22260	19743	88.69
4.	Raigad (Pen)	9929	9396	94.63
5.	Nashik (Kalwan)	40446	36717	90.78
6.	Nashik (Trimbak)	58019	52776	90.96
7.	Dhule (Taloda)	69622	66305	95.24
8.	Dhule (Nandurbar)	91588	83496	91.16
9.	Jalgaon (Yawal)	5935	5479	92.32
10.	Ahmednagar (Rajur)	13208	11486	86.96
11.	Pune (Ghodegaon)	14340	12042	83.97
12.	Nanded (Kinwat)	20288	17837	87.92
13.	Amravati (Akola)	9378	8692	92.69
14.	Amravati (Dharni)	27326	23977	87.74
15.	Nagpur (Ramtek)	15110	13718	90.79
16.	Gondia (Deori)	20090	18396	91.57
17.	Yavatmal (Pandharkawada)	36561	33562	91.79
18.	Chandrapur (Rajura)	28682	26287	91.65
19.	Chandrapur (Chimur)	11091	10165	91.65
20.	Gadchiroli (Ettapalli)	12445	11772	94.59
21.	Gadchiroli (Dhanora)	5413	4921	90.91
22.	Bhamragad	11846	10835	91.47
	Total	**634580**	**578136**	**91.11**

Table 3.5

Food Availability

Sr. No.	*Months of Food Availability*	*No. of families*	*Percentage*
1.	0 to 2 months	4 + 39 landless	35
2.	2 to 4 months	29	24
3.	4 to 6 months	23	19
4.	6 to 8 months	19	15
5.	8 to 10 months	8	6
6.	More than ten	1	1
	Total	**123**	**100**

From the above statistics, it is evident that tribal women do suffer from health and nutritional hazards due to economic, educational and social backwardness and lack of resources. Furthermore, these problems vary from tribe to tribe. Katkaris and Dhor Kolis of western Maharashtra are landless and very poor as compared to tribes having land.

BELIEFS AND PRACTICES REGARDING DELAYED DELIVERIES

A Case Study of Chenchus

Chenchus are a primitive tribe in Andhra Pradesh, Dr. P.K.Bhowmick highlights the risks and complications in his monographs regarding delivery process. Given below are details of the same.

Stoppage of periodic menstruation is taken as the first sign of pregnancy of all child-bearing women and chenchu women are no exceptions. Two or three months after stoppage of menstruation the chenchu women report it to an elderly female member of the family. In many villages the husband, however, is not informed. Informants from village Marripalem said that their wives never reveal the secret of their being pregnant to them.

There are no special ceremonies traditionally performed, except in the villages of Mannanoor and Srisaliam, is connection with conception or pregnancy. The following case study illustrates the details of the ceremonial bath performed in Mannanoor.

During her pregnancy, Yallamma's mother-in-law requested all married women of her village to attend the ceremony. An auspicious day was fixed by the village headman. Yallamma was standing in the front yard of her house and the married women one by one, applied turmeric paste on her forehead and then poured water on her head. This ceremony is called by them Neelluposukunnadi (one who has taken bath i.e. conceived). The informants could not explain the significance of this ceremony. It is an aspect of their tradition, according to them. Sweets were presented to the pregnant woman by some of the women attending the ceremony.

After bath she wore a sari presented by her brother. The same procedure has been noticed in the case of Kudumula Badamma, a resident of Srisailam village.

Vevillu or pregnancy vomitings, lack of taste for usual food, desire for foul food-stuffs, etc. start in the 3rd or 5th month of the pregnancy. This initial pregnancy condition is called *Bycala* in local parlance. It is observed by the neighbouring women and they discuss among themselves that a particular woman is Muttulappindi, which means that the particular woman is missing her menstrual cycle. Gradually, the outer symptoms of pregnancy like bulging of abdomen, heavy breasts, etc. are noticed.

Most of the expectant mothers perform day-to-day household chores in the initial stages, while during the advanced stage some of them are not allowed to do hard or heavy work, as it may cause harm to the baby in the womb. In villages like Appapurpenta and Pullaipalli, the Chenchus are a very poor lot. Consequently, the pregnant women are required to continue their routine duties. They have to assist the husband in the matter of collection of honey, fruits, tubers and other minor forest produce, even when they are in the advanced stage of pregnancy. In village Peddamanthanala, Jallinagamma was doing hard work in the usual course for the first three months. She performed only household duties at the advanced stage of pregnancy. Uttaluri Yallamma of the village Mannanoor, Uttaluri Nagamma of Byrluti had to perform routine household duties and collect minor forest produces even in the advanced stage of pregnancy. Kudumula Edamma of Srisailam performed only light domestic work like preparation of food and looking after the children. Economically well off pregnant women perform light work in their advanced stages, whereas economically poor women whose services are very essential for the maintenance of the family perform hard work.

Sexual urge diminishes during pregnancy, according to Jallipentamma and tokal Gurramma. When their husbands come to know that their wives are carrying, they too desist from expressing their sex urge, according to the above mentioned informants. But the couple may share the same bed till delivery. They do not feel the natural excitement in sexual intercourse during the pregnancy, according to Yallamma of Mannanoor. She further told that she had completely abstained herself from sexual activity from the fifth month onwards as she felt that it might be harmful to the baby in the womb if one indulged in sexual intercourse in that stage, Only four months after delivery the desire for sex is again revived normally, according to her. Nagamma of Byrluti felt sexual urge after fifth month of delivery. She did not permit sexual intercourse from eight month of her pregnancy and onwards as she felt that it was positively harmful to the fetus. After delivery, she had taken rest for six months. Villagers of Marripalem told that they continue sexual relations with their wives in the advanced stage of pregnancy also. One month after the delivery they again start sexual intercourse.

Desire for choicest meals increases at the initial stage. Some pregnant women eat pieces of charcoal, stones in the rice, tamarind, sour mangoes etc. There are no restrictions regarding diet during pregnancy. Mallapotula Chandramma of Pechcheruvu told that a pregnant woman should eat whatever she likes. Otherwise, the offspring suffers from ear disease. If the baby is found suffering from ear disease, it is attributed to the fact that the mother not eat something which was liked by her during pregnancy. To cure the disease, she has to get that desired food and eat so that her desire is fulfilled and as a result the disease will be cured. During pregnancy, the expectant mother gets cooperation and sympathetic treatment from all the members of her family.

Regarding forecasting sex of the child before its birth, the chenchus have a strong belief that pregnancy lasts for nine months in the case of a male child, and 10 months in case of a female child. It is believed that female child in the womb begs God to bless her with one month additional time for escaping from the difficulties on the earth as she has to perform so many duties throughout the day.

'Birth of a child is the blessing of God'. This is the Chenchu concept of birth. Miscarriage is considered to bring ill-luck to the family. It is also thought as a punishment given to the couple by God for a grievous sin committed by them previously. Mostly the sins of the females are considered responsible for miscarriages, according to the Chenchu informants of both sexes. Proper precautionary measures are to be taken to avert abortions.

Among the Chenchus, pregnant women have to observe the following taboos:

1. She should not go to the burial ground;
2. Both husband and wife are allowed to see the dead body, but neither the pregnant woman nor her husband should touch the dead body. Husband may go to the burial ground but he should not participate in the digging of a pit for consigning the dead body in it. He should not pour earth on the dead body. He is also not allowed to have vermilion mark on his forehead at that time. The husband is allowed to take cooked food in the house of the deceased person, whereas, the pregnant woman is not allowed to eat the cooked food in that house. Uncooked rice and meat are sent to her house. She has to cook them for herself;

3. Pregnant women should not attend on a girl in puberty. If she violates the taboo, the fetus may suffer injury resulting in abortion.

Delivery takes place either in the pregnant woman's mother's hut or in her husband's hut. If the parents of the woman are alive and could afford to maintain their daughter during pregnancy and after the child-birth, the daughter is taken to her parent's hut for delivery. Otherwise, the delivery takes place in the husband's hut. Among the Chenchus, first delivery generally takes place in the mother's house. If the delivery is arranged in husband's hut and if her parents are living in the same village, her mother comes to assist her at the time of delivery. There is a custom that the first child must be born in the mother's place and the second in the husband's place, according to some Chenchu women.

As the Chenchus have a large number of nuclear families, naturally the husband is the only man who generally stays at home at the time of advanced stage of delivery and watches the symptoms cautiously and arranges for her assistance. If she is in her mother's house, she is taken care of by her mother and sometimes by her elder sisters.

The Chenchus live in circular single-room huts. Consequently, there is practically no possibility for setting apart a confinement room. The male members, unmarried girls and children are not allowed to attend the expectant mother at the time of delivery. They are temporarily accommodated in the huts of their neighbours and come and stay in the house after delivery.

At the time of delivery, a midwife is asked to attend the pregnant woman. She is locally called Mantrasani and she belongs to Chenchu community only. In village Marripalem, there is one midwife names Bodi ankamma. Generally she is asked to assist the pregnant woman at the time of delivery. Likewise, in a villages Mannanoor, Srisailam, Pedamanthanala, Byrluti and Pothurajupenta there are Mantrasanis. In some villages no midwife is found. In such cases, the pregnant woman is assisted by her mother, mother-in-law, elder sisters and other elderly neighbouring women.

"Delivery takes place in sitting position. Chigurla Lewelamma came to her mother's house for her first delivery. Her eldest sister Nallapotula Chandramma had also come from Hyderabad where she is living to attend her sister's delivery; Leelamma was directed to catch hold of a cloth which was tied to the roof of the house for affording support in a sitting posture. The mother sat on the backside to support the woman in delivery. The services of midwife were not requisitioned in this case".

If the delivery is difficult, they seek the help of the medicine man. In village Marripalem, there is one medicine man that belongs to the Chenchu community. The husband requisitions his services if the expectant woman is thought to be possessed by evil spirit. There is a belief among the Chenchus that difficult delivery is caused by the wrath of some angered deity. After his arrival, the medicine-man catches hold of her hands and makes a sort of performance to ascertain whether the woman is possessed by an evil spirit or not and finally identifies the name of the deity responsible for the difficult labour. After identifying the deity, her husband is asked to perform worship of that deity for affording easy delivery to his wife. The husband also takes a vow to perform worship to that deity if that woman delivers the child without difficulty. The husband fulfils the vow after she delivers the child.

There is also another practice for affording an easy delivery according to the informants from Marripalem village. All the men, women and children stand in a line from the expectant mother's house up to the well. The person who stands near the well collects some water in a Chembu (a small water vessel) from the well and that vessel containing water is passed from one to the other in the line. Finally, the person who stands near the woman in labour hands over the vessel with water to her. The reason behind this practice is that there may be some sacred people among those who stand in the line. The water carried by them may also become sacred by the touch of those sacred persons. Drinking of this sacred water by the woman in labour may ensure easy delivery. If the case is still serious, then only the services of a doctor are commissioned.

Delivery is locally known as Theeradhamaduta, literally meaning taking the bath. After the birth of the child, the mother and the child are cleaned by the midwife with a piece of cloth dipped in hot water. The delivery place is also cleaned by her. She keeps the baby on a piece of cloth beside its mother lying on the mat. The mother of the child drinks country liquor after delivery for relief from the painful after-efforts. No other medicine is used for this purpose. All the persons who assemble there at the time of delivery demand liquor from the husband. After drinking the liquor they all go to their respective houses.

Midwife or an elderly woman cuts the umbilical cord with a sharp edged arrow or iron-sickle (Kodavali) or knife. Sometimes a thread is used to cut the umbilical cord. It is cut 2"to 3"above the naval region.

After birth of the child, the placenta generally comes out. If the delivery occurs in the day time, the midwife or some other woman presses the abdomen of the new mother from upper to lower direction so that the after-birth condition is eased out without delay. In case of further delay, the midwife inserts her fingers into the womb for the removal of the placenta. After-birth waste matter is called Parupu in local parlance. It is put in some ashes kept in a pot and is carried by the midwife followed by the husband. The husband digs a pit by the side of his hut and buried the Parupu. In the absence of a midwife, the mother of the woman who delivered or the mother-in-law or any other close relative performs the same function.

Turmeric powder is applied at the naval region of the baby until it dries up properly. Sometimes a piece of cloth, burnt to ashes and mixed with castor oil, is applied to the remaining stub of the umbilical cord for early healing. Now-a-days, they are freely using boric acid with bandage, which is locally, knows as *Boddumamudu*. It is supplied by the women welfare centre in Byrluti (Chandrasekhar 1965:21). The head of the baby is applied with castor oil and covered with a piece of cloth. Sometimes they keep onions in the ears of the baby and tie a piece of cloth around its head to prevent ear diseases.

The midwife is required to stay for sometime after delivery for assisting the new mother and for nursing the child. She is given cooked food daily. She collects remuneration for her services. The remuneration varies from village to village. Table 3.6 shows the period of her stay and the remunerations of her services in different villages.

Table 3.6

Particulars of Midwife

Sr. No.	*Village*	*No. of days attended*	*Remuneration*	
			Cash (Rupees)	*Kind*
1.	Mannanoor	3-9 days	4/-	Liquor, food
2.	Srisailam	3 days	10/-	Liquor, new saree, blouse and meals
3.	Pedamanthanala	9-10 days	3/-	Food, liquor
4.	Byrluti	5 days	3/-	Food, liquor
5.	Pothurajupenta	3 days	5/-	Liquor
6.	Marripalem	7 days	5/-	Food, liquor

Generally a midwife stays throughout the pollution period which varies from village to village.

After delivery bleeding continues for a few days. It depends on the state of health of the mother. This period is treated as pollution period which is observed for 5 to 10 days in different villages. During this period, the mother is not allowed to move about in her place and should not touch anything or anybody. Only her assistant may touch her. She is not allowed to lie with her husband and she does not participate in any religious ceremony. She lies down all alone with the new born baby. Food is served to her in a leaf or in a separate plate. Nattapotula Chandramma of Pechcheruvu said that the new mother should not touch the fire and desecrate it. If she does so, the baby may suffer from a disease called Aggibobbalu. The same belief was in vogue in some other villages also.

During and after pollution period, the lactating mother may have to observe some restrictions regarding her diet for some time. Chicken, gourd, eggs, and meat of the rabbit were forbidden for the lactating women, as it is considered very dangerous to the health of the baby and the mother. She can eat the meat of goat, sheep and some particular vegetables. In villages Appapurpenta and Pullaipalli, the new mother regularly eats Arvaiu (a local preparation made with garlic, pepper, dried ginger, asafetida (Inguva) powder and roasted chili powder mixed with oil, mainly with rice for 3 to 10 days twice days. In Mannanoor, they take this type of food for 10 to 30 days. The body of the mother is believed to gradually dry up by eating the above mentioned food. There is no restriction for drinking liquor. In village Marripalem, the motakes takes Sankatam made from ground Jowar (Millet) and Onion Karam (onion and chili powder) with a little salt. This diet is prescribed strictly for 5 days. Nallapotula Leelamma of Pechcheruvu took hot rice and hot water without salt for 5 days. She was given a mug of hot water daily. She should not eat or drink in excess of this.

After the stoppage of blood discharge, the mother takes bath. She is applied with turmeric powder and ground nut or coconut oil all over her body, except head on that day. The midwife of mother or mother-in-law or friends attends the formal purificatory bath. There is no special ceremony associated with it. In village Pechcheruvu, Leelamma took head bath. Some leaves called Takkela, Vepa, Vayala (all forest leaves) were boiled in water until foam was formed and the water turned to green colour. This foam was applied to her head and the boiled leaves to her body. The women informants of Marripalem told that they take bath with Chamuru (butter or ghee).

The midwife washes the baby daily. In her absence, the child's grand-mother does baby's washing. They wash the baby for three months at the same spot. The child is given honey and a little water till it is able to suck the breast-milk. After 2 to 5 days of delivery, milk appears in the breasts of the mother. However, it depends on the mother's health. In individual cases, the suckling period varies from 1 year to 5 years, till the next baby is born. If the mother has no milk to feed the baby, she eats fish and crab curry for 2 to 3 days to remedy the position. After delivery, the mother takes rest for sometime. The resting period varies from 1 to 4 months, depending upon the health of the mother. Generally, she takes rest till she recoups her normal physical strength.

Prolonged and protracted labour pain is immediately cured by rubbing and pressing of the abdomen by the midwife. In case of further difficulty, supernatural potentialities are suspected to cause such trouble. In such cases, a promise is generally made in the form of vow, through appeals and prayers. After successful delivery, the name of the child is given after the name of the deity, who supposedly caused the trouble, by performing the ceremonies as promised.

According to the Census of India 1961, Vol. I "... it is found that certain magico-religious beliefs are associated with the name-giving ceremony. Magical treatment is also done if the child begins to cry, does not suckle milk properly and does not play cheerfully'.

Given the above background, it is clear that tribals have their own perceptions regarding conception, growth of foetus, delivery process, complications during pregnancy, delivery and post delivery etc. that, their perceptions and practices differ from the scientific rationale and hence the need of health education and sensitisation for safe and effective practices is need of the hour.

4

Body Image, Human Reproduction and Birth Control Practices Among the Thakars

BRIEF ETHNOGRAPHIC PROFILE OF THAKARS

The Thakars are one of the major tribes of Maharashtra, chiefly found in Raigad, Thane, Nashik, Pune and Ahmednagar districts. A few have also migrated to other districts in search of jobs.

Sub-tribes

The sub-tribes of Thakars are known as Ma Thakar and Ka Thakar respectively. The members of Thakar do not marry Ka Thakars.

Population

According to 2001 census, the total population of Thakars in Maharashtra is 4,87,696.

Physical Features

The Thakars are a small squat tribe, certainly better looking than their neighbours the Katkaris. Most Thakars are of medium height, their general complexion is brown. Hair is generally straight and wavy. They have large though not very prominent cheek bones, rather full lips and deep sunken eyes.

A diminish or marginal type of epicanthic fold. The Thakar women are noted for their bulging stomachs. They tie their saris very tightly below their navel.

Dressing Pattern

Thakar men wear a loin-cloth and occasionally a waist cloth and a blanket draped on the shoulder and a piece of cloth around their heads. Some wear a traditional type of sleeve shirt known as *'bandi'*. The women wear *'lugdi'* (Sari) very tightly wrapped around their waist, so as to leave while the Ka Thakar women have a separate *'lugadi'* (Sari) piece tucked at their waist, which is drawn over their head. Thakar women wear a blouse called *'choli'*.

Settlement Pattern

The Thakar lives or rather seems to live aloof. His preference for jungle life is the cause. A Thakar settlement is popularly known as Thakarwadi. The hamlets of Thakars are known by their clan names, names of trees, deities, etc. Some of the examples are Lobhiewadi (Clan name), Borwadi (Fruit name), Nagyachiwadi (Deity name), etc.

Economic Life

The economic position of a Thakar is determined by the amount of grain he holds, number of ploughs, live stock and size of the house he owns. They are small scale cultivators and grow rice, *nagli, vasi,* one or two pulses and few vegetables. The tribesmen are busy in cultivation from June to October. From November to May they are either busy in minor forest collection, fishing, hunting or doing daily wage labour. Some of the educated Thakar youth have taken up jobs in Government and private firms.

Family Life

A family is usually formed of a man who is the head of the family, his wife and children. Married daughters must live with their husbands, since the family types of Thakar society are patriarchal, patrilineal and patrilocal. Married son either continues to live with the father, or gets separated and makes a new home. Married brothers do not live together. Both joint and nuclear family types are prevalent among the Thakars.

Marriage

Marriage is one of the most important events in the life of a Thakar. Preparation for it starts with the selection of a bride. There are certain Kuli (Clans) or families which cannot intermarry, e.g. the Padirs cannot marry Padirs, but can marry Parthis. Age at marriage for the boys is 16-20 and girls 14-18.

Having approved of the bride in the preliminary talks, the settlement is ratified by the ceremony of betrothal which is called *supari phodane*. The action is symbolic of finalising marital relationship to proceed with further ceremonies. Marriage usually takes place at the brides' house. Dej or bride price is both in cash and kind to the girls' parents by the boys' parents. Monogamy is the most common form of marriage among the Thakars.

Religion

The Thakar supernatural beliefs are mainly expressed in ritual and magical practices. His pantheon consists of a number of deities. Among them are the village gods whose names are as follows: *Chedhoba, Vaghoba, Khambya, Bhairi,* etc. The *Hirva* represents peacock from the animal world. *Murya, Khais, Vetal and Hadal* comes from the spirit world. *Virdev* and *Supali* represents the ancestors. *Kanisdev* is yet another God of Ear, who appears when a patient suffers from severe earache.

Sun is the most powerful of all Gods and mother earth is his wife. Moon is his brother and water again has brotherly relationship with sun and moon. The lightening and *holi* (festival of fire and goddess of fertility)/The *Satvai* (mother earth) is the goddess fortune and fertility. Their religion shows animistic traits.

Birth Rituals

When a woman feels her time is near, she goes home, changes her sari, wraps a piece of cloth around her loins and his down supine on a rough blanket in the inner chamber resting her head on a folded cloth. She is assisted and attended by a *suine* (midwife) and *potdhari* (*suine's* helpmate). If there is much delay or the delivery is difficult, charmed ash is brought from a *Bhagat* and applied on the forehead of the parturient woman. Another measure is to wet a part of her husband's loin cloth in a little water and give the water to the ailing woman to drink. Placing herbs such as a plantain (Musa paradisica) roots and/or the root of a milk weed called *rui* (calotropis gigante) are placed on the nape of the neck and are supposed to be efficacious.

The delivery posture is east-west, with the mother's head pointing towards east while her vaginal opening pointing towards the west. The Thakars believe that the mother earth (*Dantari*) who is towards the west must see the child first. Mother earth the wife of sun bestows fortune and life on every newborn.

The midwife uses a sickle (*koyati*) to cut the umbilical cord (*nal*). The cord is buried outside the western wall of the house. This is done to prevent it from an object of witchcraft in order to harm the new born. On the fifth day after the birth of the newborn the Thakars perform the ritual of Sati. The midwife worships the goddess of fertility and fortune (*dantari*-mother earth) by thanking her. The midwife gets liquor, a hen or a coconut or blouse along with the same cash of Rs. 50/- to Rs. 100/- of late. Earlier they would take Rs.5/- only.

Death Rituals

The Thakars have elaborate rituals which are carried out after death. The dead person is placed on the floor with the head pointing south. The dead are buried by the Thakars.

On the tenth day in case of married males, ninth day in case of married females and seventh day in case of a bachelor or spinster, the ritual of soul migration is performed to send his or her soul to heaven.

In his book captioned. "Medical World of Tribals", Tribhuwan Robin (1998) has given in detail the symbols and meanings associated with soul migration rituals of the Thakars.

Body Image—Perceptions

A Thakar's knowledge of human body is based on the close observation and his study of animal and plant life in and around the forest. His ideas about the anatomy and physiology of human body are derived from what he knows about the animals he kills for food. His interpretation of human body on the whole reflects his ideology about universe. Khanda sarkha panda – meaning the human body is nothing but the image of cosmos. (Tribhuvan Robin 1998:163).

Chaphekar L.N. (1961:83) highlights the perception of Thakars as far as main bodily organs. According to the Thakars the body of the beast has following main organs:

1. *Kalij* (liver)
2. *Phuphus* (lungs)
3. *Dil* (heart)
4. *Pitta* (bile)
5. *Atadi* (intestines)
6. *Potala* (stomach)
7. *Yir* (neck)
8. *Mutlani* (urinary bladder)
9. *Satputi* (duodenum)

Chaphekar (1961) also documented a song which describes some anatomical and physiological aspects of human body in a question and answer form. The song is known as *Deha Bhangadre Gane* – Songs concerned with human body.

TRADITIONAL CONTRACEPTIVE PRACTICES AMONG THAKARS

While working with 400 tribal medical practitioners including Thakars, Katkaris, Mahadev Kolis and Warlis, Dr Tribhuvan (1998) observed that the medical practitioners give medicines to prevent pregnancies, for abortion, for increasing semen production and so on. It was at this point of time i.e.

during 1990 to 1993; Tribhuvan (ibid) discovered that tribals do have traditional contraceptive beliefs and practices. Some of the beliefs and practices of traditional contraception are as follows:

Observe sex taboos: One of the most common techniques practiced by the Thakars is to refrain from having sex with the wife from 10th to 17th day after her menstrual cycle. They believe that sexual intercourse during these days can initiate pregnancy.

Use of cloth: Even if the couple has sex from 10th to 17th day after the menstrual period, they keep a cloth on the vagina to avoid semen getting in it.

Removing the Penis / Coitus Interruptus: Some males expressed that they penetrate the penis inside the vagina during the intercourse, but remove it out before they release the semen. In doing so the semen does not get in to the vagina, thus preventing the pregnancy.

Community approved sex prevention taboos: Thakars are aware of the co-relation between family size and income. If a man has more than seven to eight children, there are cultural provisions to socially control them. One such ritual is documented by Tribhuvan Robin (1998) is as follows:

BODY IMAGE: THAKAR PERCEPTION

(a) Difference Between Males and Females

According to Thakar belief system, the difference between males and females is spelt out on the basis of absence and presence of certain bodily organs. The table given next page reveals the same.

Nature and role of medical practitioners: Medical practitioners certainly play an important role in educating their tribesmen about body image, diagnosis and therapy. They are health care providers for the tribals. Their role in health education according to us is certainly of great significance. Efforts should be made to train their medical practitioners, give them incentives in kind and cash keeping the local traditions in view.

Difference between males and females: Thakar perceptions:

Sr. No.	*Indicators*	*Males*	*Females*
1.	Testicles	Males have testicles	Females do not
2.	Urethra	Males have it	Females do not
3.	Beard and moustache	Males have it	Females do not
4.	Deep voice	Males have it	Females do not
5.	Breasts	Males don't have it	Females have breasts
6.	Long hair	Males don't have it	Females have long hair
7.	Delicate body	Males don't have it	Females have a delicate body
8.	Pregnancy	Males do not experience pregnancy	Females experience pregnancy
9.	Strength	Males are stronger	Females are weaker
10.	Eating capacity	Males eat more	Females eat less
11.	Ability to bear pain	Males cannot bear pain	Females do deliver children
12.	Nipples	Males do not have prominent nipples	Females have nipples and have breast milk.

From the qualitative data on Thakar perception of body image and traditional contraceptive beliefs and practices among the Thakars, it is clear that their perceptions, beliefs and practices are deeply rooted in their culture. Their beliefs and practices are hence intertwined with their symbolic systems and they are associated with cultural meanings.

Health policy makers and health educators who have allopathic and administrative background tend to ignore the socio-cultural, symbolic and psychological aspect of tribal health. It is therefore, necessary to tackle tribal health case and services issues from an inter-disciplinary angle. We certainly advocate the role of social scientists in primary health care in India.

(b) Openings of the Body

The Song Questions

In our body oh brother
Where is the bone sixteen cubits?

To our body oh brother
How many doors are there?

In our body oh brother
Which part is a cubit and quarter?

In our body oh brother
Where if the secret fire that ever burns?

In our body oh brother
Which is the small bone

In our body oh brother
Where is the 'Vithal vein'?

In our body oh brother
Where is the flowing Ganges?
In our body oh brother
Where lies the dry ocean?

There are problems oh brother
Please explain me oh brother

The Answers

The bone sixteen cubit long is the
Vein of our body oh brother

In our body oh brother
There are nine doors oh brother

The place a cubit and a quarter long
Is the circumference of our head

In our body oh brother to the left
is the second fire that burns

To the bone as small as sesame
Is in our penis, oh brother

And the vital vein oh brother
Is our throat oh brother

And the dry ocean is our
Throat oh brother

At another village Chaphekar reported a different version about the Doors of human body (1961: 82)

To our body, oh brother,
How many doors are there?
There are ten doors oh brother
How many are open?
Nine are open oh brother
And the tenth one is secret.

Chaphekar (1961:82), further points out that the 'sacred door' is supposed to be the apex of the scalp. The song continues to say that the key to the sacred door is with the *Sadguru*, the spiritual teacher and opens the door when the leaves the body.

Chaphekar's brief account on the Thakars ideology of body image was an incentive for the researcher to probe into their concept of body symbolism and ethno-physiology from an emic perspective. Interpretations regarding how the body functions, what makes it exist, what fluids and elements does it constitute, how the various systems of the body function, their concept of life and a detailed analysis of body symbolism is discussed in this chapter.

(c) Bodily Fluids

A Thakar classifies human bodily fluids in to two categories, namely:

- *The fluid of life:* meaning the fluids such as water, blood, breast milk, sperms, vaginal fluid, which sustain and create life;
- *Excretory fluids:* fluids such as urine, sweat, menstrual blood, tears, pus, mucus etc. that are excreted or thrown out by the body fall in the second category. Their knowledge of both fluids of life and excretory fluids is vast. They interpret healthy and unhealthy conditions of the human body based on the colour, production, type, the contribution of these fluids to the body, symbolic aspects of the bodily fluids and so on. The Thakar's knowledge of the above said categories of bodily fluids was assessed in the light of health and behavioural aspects.

(i) The Fluids of Life

Fluids of life according to the Thakars have two types of functions:

(a) Fluids that create life

(b) Fluids that nourish and sustain life.

The Thakars believe that sperms (*Virya*) are stocked in the forehead, just above the fronto-nasal suture. Sperms are produced by two worms (*Kidas*) which are situated in the forehead. During the sexual intercourse these sperms travel down from the forehead touching the *atma* (soul) which is situated below the sternum and comes out through the urethra. Presence of testes is just a sign of being a male species. (Chaphekar 1960).

The Thakars believes that 40 morsels (*ghas*) of food produces 1/2 ml of semen and just one small speck or drop of it fertilises the flower (egg-cell) of the female. Just as the flower produces fruit, so also a woman liberates flowers which are stocked in her worms of forehead and produces a child.

This concept of reproduction, very much resembles plants. In plants pollen grains fall on the stigma and fertilise and hence a fruit is produced. A woman liberates a flower which is fertilised just by one drop of semen and therefore child (fruit) is produced.

A sterile/barren woman does not liberate 'flower' (in this case egg cell). A man whose semen colour is yellow is believed to be sterile. The status of both sterile men and women in the Thakar society is very low. They are prohibited from participating in fertility rituals such as puberty rite, wedding, turmeric ceremony, *panchvi punjan* (worship of mother Earth) and so on.

Thus semen and vaginal fluids are the main sources of producing life. The combination of these two results into an offspring and therefore they are classified as life fluids that contribute in creating life.

(ii) Fluids that Sustain Life

Blood, breast milk and water are some of the major fluids which according to Thakars sustain life. Their perceptions of these major fluids revealed following facts:

Blood

Blood (*Raghat*) is the most important fluid in the human body that contributes to its survival. Blood contributes to the production of breast milk, sperms, vaginal fluid and strength. They judge a person's strength and stage of growth; ill health conditions based on the colour of his/her blood. The table given on next page shows their concept of colour symbolism associated with human blood.

Blood according to the Thakars must be utilised by doing work so as to dispose it in the form of energy. It should be utilised for the production of breast milk, semen, vaginal fluid etc. but never must be accumulated in the body. A person who does not work hard accumulates blood in the body and invites diseases (*rog*). Blood circulates in the body in an anti-clockwise manner (the auspicious manner). The Thakars believe sun, moon, clouds, winds etc. move in an auspicious direction. Hence air, *agni* (fire), water (*pani*), blood (*raghat*), (*tej*) move in an anti-clockwise fashion.

Table 4.1

Concepts of Blood Colour and Illness

Sr. No.	*Colour of Blood*	*Concepts*
1.	Red Blood	a. Children and teenagers have red blood. b. Red blood is a sign of healthy body. c. It also symbolises power or strength a child or teenager has which is fairly good.
2.	Reddish Orange	a. Adults have reddish orange blood. b. Symbolises higher degree of strength. c. Sign of healthy body.
3.	Black Colour	a. Old people have black colour blood. b. Symbolises lowest degree of strength. c. Sign of ill health.
4.	Reddish black	a. Menstruating women have this blood. b. It is hot in nature and has a foul smell. c. Is evil and brings about diseases such as leprosy, Sexually Transmitted Diseases etc.
5.	Yellow	Yellow colour blood in some parts such as eyes, nails and if seen on the skin is a sign of Jaundice Blood which turns into yellowish green colour is 'pus' again a sign of ill health.
6.	Greenish Yellow	Leprosy patients are believed to have this colour. When they die they are cremated and the smoke that comes out is greenish yellow colour.
7.	Bluish colour	When a person is bitten by a cobra his/her blood turns bluish in colour because of the effect of poison. It's a signal of death.
8.	White	White discharge among the women is considered to be a sign of ill health as it is against the orderly routine of menstrual flow.

All the *Dayan jatis* (evil social groups), including the Mahars, Mangs, Chamars, Thakars, Kathkaris etc. believe that anti-clockwise movement is an auspicious movement. While the *Dev jatis* (god) like Brahmans, Marathas, Kunbis, Mahadev kolis, Gujratis etc. believe that clockwise movement is auspicious and anti-clockwise is inauspicious. Thus all auspicious rites performed in the *Davan* (evil) jati show anti-clockwise movements or actions while it is exactly opposite with the *dev* (godlike) jatis.

Breast Milk

The belief that breast milk is produced from women's blood in her breast is a very common belief among the Thakars. An infant survives on breast milk nearly for a year. Milk of a mother is a medium through which her strength (blood) is passed on to the child. Yet another phenomena regarding breast milk which is directly connected with the child's health is their concept of '*Naska Dudh*' (spoilt milk).

The Thakars believe that mothers do not breast feed the child for the first five days. They believe that the mother's milk is thick and is harmful as it causes indigestion in the child. The word '*Naska*' means spoilt. For nine months and nine days the fetus is in the mother's womb and the mother's body internally gets polluted with spermatic (sticky) effect due to menstrual blood which according to the Thakars is evil. Due to the thickness of menstrual blood which is inside the body for nine months and the spermatic effect the normal blood of the women also gets slightly thick and hence cheesed milk or 'Colostrum milk' (spoilt milk) is produced. For five days the colostrum milk is squeezed out and the child is given goat's milk, honey and water.

Water: The King of Bodily Fluids

The source of life giving fluids is water. Thakars believe that blood, breast milk, vaginal fluid, mucus, sweat, semen, pus, tears, urine etc. are produced because of intake of water. Blood is of course produced as a result of water and food together, which turns into juice which is acted upon by *agni* (heat) in the stomach and then converted into blood. The human body has life only because of intake of water and food. Even the *atma* (soul) which is situated just below the sternum is nourished by water, wind, fire and light.

Thus, whatever water and food is taken in it contributes to the production of blood first – blood then turns into breast milk. Vaginal fluid and semen are produced in the respective worms (kidas) of males and females in their foreheads.

Water is considered as God. Water is believed to be the brother of Sun and Moon. Therefore water is used in many auspicious occasions by the Thakars like healing rites, marriage, turmeric ceremony rites, purification rites, fertility rites and so on. Water is very scarce in Karjat tribal areas. The tribals have hard times during summer. Most Thakars do not use water after defecation. They use stones or leaves. They believe that it is an insult to their God and his brothers Sun and Moon.

Excretory Fluids

Fluids such as urine, sweat, tears, mucus, pus etc. are believed to be residual fluids of water. Water and food which is consumed gets converted to blood and waste products such as urine and excreta. Fluids such as pus and menstrual blood are spoilt produced of good blood and hence are eliminated out of the body naturally. Tears are produced in the eyes. Mucus is believed to be the excreta of worms (*Kidas*) which are situated just above the fronto-nasal suture.

The state of health and ill health is judged on the colour and abnormality of the excretory fluids. Thus when mucus is very watery it is believed that the forehead has been overexposed to cold water and wind. When the colour of urine changes to yellow or red it is a sign of ill health.

The Thakars believe that if a person walks or works in the Sun (heat) for a long time his blood gets burnt and comes out of his body in the form of sweat (*gham*). To substitute the loss of blood one needs to then take water. One feels thirsty and drinks more water which again turns into blood and blood into sweat. The movement of these fluids in the body and their elimination is done with the help of wind in the body. Blood circulation in the body is because of the flow of wind in the body.

(d) Physiology of Bodily Systems

Indigenous knowledge of body physiology very much differs from the scientific knowledge of the physiology of various bodily systems, namely, respiratory system, circulatory system, and nervous system and so on. The science of ethno-physiology as a sub-discipline of medical Anthropology deals with beliefs, values, perceptions, knowledge and understanding of a community regarding the functioning of various bodily systems and organs and their contribution to body survival.

It is very necessary to understand people's concept of body physiology, dietary behaviour, illness etiology, ethno-medical therapy, preventive medicine, etc. in order to implement culturally acceptable health education programmes.

Nitcher and Nitcher (1981:75) have pointed out that the elaborate and detailed belief systems and underlying food habits in traditional societies are often overlooked. Sometimes they are dismissed as unrelated and haphazard collection of superstitions and customs based on ignorance.

Today especially in a developing country like India where 80 per cent of the population resides in the rural and tribal areas food traditions and related concepts of ethno-physiology still continue to play an integral part of many societies. They often help to maintain cultural identity and traditional values in the face of destabilising influences.

In order to educate people on health it is very necessary to understand what they have. Study their belief system and build on what is available. The Thakar concept of ethno-physiology of bodily systems reveals following facts:

(e) Concept of Reproduction

Thakars' concepts of reproduction resemble the plants. Just as a plant produces fruit from a flower after having fertilised by water, so also human beings both male and female produce an offspring (fruit) after sexual intercourse.

Semen according to the Thakars is stocked in the forehead. In the forehead i. e. just above the fronto-nasal stature dwell the 'worms of life' (*kidas*) which produce semen. Thus sperms as believed by Thakars are liberated from these *kidas* and come out through the urethra touching the soul (*atma*), carrying the element of life with it. One drop of sperm fertilises a flower (*phool*) which is liberated by a woman's 'worms' from the forehead and come out in the from of vaginal fluid in the vagina, where a drop of sperm fertilises it and is nurtured into a fruit (fetus) into the mother's womb. Thus, if two flowers are released by a woman during sexual intercourse and if they are fertilised by two drops of sperms twins are born.

The Thakars believe that for nine months and nine days a pregnant woman does not menstruate. The fetus lives on her menstrual blood. Besides this the fetus gets sufficient warmth, air, water, blood, light etc. from the mother's body. Thakars' concept of reproduction is thus symbolic and expresses the natural fertilisation concepts which they observe in plants.

(f) Concept of Digestion

Digestion of food according to Thakars starts in the mouth where food is ground and pushed in the stomach *(potali)* with the help of wind. In the stomach fire (heat), light, water converts the food into liquid from. This liquid food is filtered and separated into blood and excreta in the intestines. Excreta comes out from the anus *(Gupt Darwaza* or secret door), spoilt water (urine) comes out from urethral/vaginal opening.

The Thakars believe that for digestion of two *bhakars* (coarse bread) two glasses of water are required, if one *bhakar* is consumed on must drink one glass of water. The proportion should be equal. Bread *(Bhakar)* prepared from wheat or *bajra* (millet) needs more water for digestion as they are believed to be heavy. Thus one *bhakar* of *bajra* requires 2 ½ glasses of water. On enquiring from a Thakar what happens when one doesn't drink water after food. The reply was 'stomach upset'. No water, no digestion. Overeating, wrong combination of foods, too hot or cold foods cause indigestion.

The digestive power of an adult and a youth is greater than a child and an old person. The ability to digest food varies at different ages. It takes at least 3 hours for food to be digested to blood. Food helps body to grow and survive.

(g) Concept of Respiration

Thakars believe that air is one of the most important constituents of the human body. It is inhaled from the atmosphere and circulated in different parts of the body by the *phuphus* (lungs). Air in the body contributes to circulation and digestion processes. The concept of oxygen and its role etc is absent among Thakar's. They classify auspicious and inauspicious air (*vara*). The auspicious air is one that flows from east to west and from north to south. Human beings breathe air from North, West and East. The air or wind flowing from South is inauspicious and caused illness and brings about death. South is the direction of death and evil. While east is from where rises the Sun, the creator, west, the direction of mother earth and north, the dwelling place of Gods.

(h) Concept of Nervous System

Atma (soul) is the seat of thinking. It is situated right below the sternum in a cage of ribs. Human brain is termed as '*mun*' which also helps to think but all sensory actions are coordinated by the *atma*. Most informants said that all nerves are linked with the *atma*. A bad *atma* allows bad thoughts to enter human body and vice versa.

Nerves are attached to muscles and bones and hence make the body flexible. Movement of body is possible because of nerves. Thus all biological actions of desire for having sex, food, water etc. is governed by the *atma* (soul).

The Thakar's concept of excretion to certain extent resembles to the 'foreign matter theory' of Louis Kunhey – a Naturopath. They believe that unutilized and waste mater in the body must be eliminated through excretion, blood letting, surgery, suction methods etc. The presence of waste matter in the body causes diseases. Efforts must be made to eliminate these matters. Of course their interpretation is not that scientific as Kunhey's. They do believe in elimination of waste products from the body.

Thus sweat, excreta, urine, menstrual blood, spoilt blood, mucus etc are waste products that the body throws out. Sweat is thrown out through skin, excreta by anus, spoilt blood by blood letting and through natural menstrual flow.

(i) Circulatory System Concepts

The Thakar's believe that blood is circulated in the body in an anti-clock manner with the help of wind (*vara*) that is present in the body. The anti-clock movement of blood is associated with movement of cosmic objects such as sun, moon, clouds etc. Anti-clock movement of blood is a symbol of auspicious movement in this context. Blood is situated in veins (*nadya*). While a person is sleeping, the blood keeps on circulating.

Atma (Soul): The Co-ordinator of all bodily systems:

Atma (soul) of a human being is situated just below the sternum according to the Thakar's. It is associated with life (*jeev*) of a person. It exists in the human body, to keep a person alive depending on the number of days destined by mother earth, who writes the life span of a child after its birth on its forehead.

Atma according to Thakar constitutes fire (*agni*), water (*pani*), wind (*vara*) and light (*tej*). It is situated in the cage of ribs. It gets light and fire from the sun and moon, wind from the cosmos and water from man. Thus an *atma* needs a regular flow of water, light, fire and wind which it gets from cosmos. A person is alive because *atma* dwells in him.

A Thakar song on the *atma* goes on to state:

Pinjara Banivala Patichare
Aatmadhi Ragho Motyachare
Pinjara Akashi Dulere
Aatmandhi Ragho Bolere
Pinjara Gela Ununire
Raghoba Gela Udunire
Gela Swargachya Vatire
Tethe Anandachi Madire
Tyachi Annandi Madire

The translation of the song

In the cage of flexible sticks
There dwells the parrot,

The parrot speaks sweetly
As the case swings in the sky

It so happened oh brother
The cage was broken
And as the cage broke away
The parrot got ready to fly away
He flew towards heaven
Where exists a place of happiness.

Meaning of the Song

About seven to eight Thakar's who were singing this song during a healing ritual were asked to provide with the meaning of the song. They explained that the cage symbolises the ribs of the human being. In which dwells the *atma* or soul (parrot). Every cage breaks some or the other time in life. Breaking of the cage symbolises death. The parrot flies away, meaning the soul leaves human body for heaven where always happiness reigns.

On enquiring from the respondents, how does a soul leave human body? They said, we get to know of this by looking at the corpse. If the mouth of the dead body is open it means that the *atma* has left the body through the mouth. So is the case if eyes are open. If both eyes and mouth are closed the Thakar's believe that the *atma* has left the person's body either through ears or nose or through the scalp of the apex as reported by Chaphekar (1961:82).

On the ninth day, in case of married women, tenth day in case of married men and seventh day in case of bachelors and spinsters after their death the Thakars perform the ritual of soul migration. The aim of the ritual is to send the sould of the dead person to heaven. A *palas* leaf (*butea monosperma*) is taken on which a stone studded in rice flour is placed and ritually left in the water along with nine other flour balls with no stone in them.

The leaf symbolises the body of the dead person, the rice flour ball the cage and the stone (*jeev khada*) symbolises the soul of the dead person which is left in a running river water facing the east for it is to merge with the cosmos and go back to heaven which is towards the east. The other nine rice flour balls symbolise the ten bodily openings in which dwell the planetary spirits. These are also left in the water to merge with the cosmos.

A Thakar riddle goes on to say '*Manev pind banavito_pun parmatma atma banavito*', meaning man makes the body (fetus), but the soul (*atma*) is the foetus is created by 'Sun God'. *Atma* according to the Thakars is the coordinator of all the systems of the body and controls all the physiological and nervous functions of the body. What the human body symbolises in different ritual healing contexts or situations is explained in the second part of the chapter.

(j) Human Body as a Natural Symbol

The Thakars associate their body morphology, anatomy and physiology to that of a tree. It is their belief that the human body is very much similar to the natural elements which a plant comprises of.

Bones: The skeletal framework of the human body is associated with the trunk and branches of the tree.

Flesh and Skin: The flesh and skin of the human body is associated with the bark (covering of the trunk and branches).

Blood: This red fluid in the human body is associated with the sap, the latex and/or water content in the tree.

Soul (Atma): The human beings have soul (*atma*) which is situated just below the sternum so also the trees have *atma* in the roots. The *atma* is believed to be the seat of intelligence and co-ordinates all the systems and also controls the thinking process. There is no concept of nervous system.

Veins / Arteries: The human body have blood vessels like arteries, veins and capillaries which are a part of the circulatory system. In a similar manner the *atma* of the tree which is present in the roots pumps the water and food to all the parts of the plant body through the vascular tissues xylem and phloem.

Hair: Just as human beings have hair on their body so also the plants have hair on the leaves, branches and on trunks, according to the Thakar's.

Feelings: Akin to human beings plants also have feelings and emotions and are hurt/wounded when they are cut.

(k) Concept of Death

Plants die or are killed when they are uprooted or destroyed from the roots. This is similar to the human body which becomes a corpse once the *atma*/soul leaves it.

Human body and plant body becomes mud after their death: Both the human and plant body after their death return back to the earth and turn into mud. Human body: (*Pind*).

Reproductive System: The flowers of the trees are turned into fruit after fertilisation. The female reproductive organ of the tree is its flower and the male reproductive organ is the water. The water drop (fertile water) from the *atma* situated in the roots fertilizes every flower of the tree which bears fruit.

(l) Male and Female Reproductive System

The Thakar's differentiate between a male and a female on the presence of testicles among the males and breasts among the females. The Thakars believe that males have two worms (*kidas*), white in colour present in the head above the fronto-nasal suture and when the *kidas* excrete mucus flows out of the nose.

If a person drinks liquor, he becomes intoxicated and loses his balance. An intoxicating drink makes the *kidas* swirl due to which the person feels giddy and loses his balance.

A person is believed to suffer from a headache when these worms (*kidas*) start biting the brain. The *kidas* are also believed to have a reproductive function. The *kidas* produce sperms which flow down from the head during intercourse and flow out of the penis. One drop of semen is capable of fertilising a flower which is produced by the female *kidas* and also flows down during intercourse.

Sperm (water) + Flower (egg) = Child (fruit)

When two flowers are contributed by the female *kidas*, these flowers are fertilised by two drops of sperms and results in twins.

2 flowers + 2 drops of sperms = twins.

3 flowers + 3 drops of sperms = triplets.

4 flowers + 4 drops of sperms = quadruplets.

It is believed (by the Thakar's) that the flower (egg contributed by the woman) opens up and receives the sperm drop to produce the fruit (child). Flowers are produced in a woman after menstruation.

Classification of Male / Female aspects among plants and its significance: The Thakar's have a peculiar fashion of differentiating male from female plants. Some plants and trees are given male and female status and have integral socio-cultural meaningful functions within the Thakar's culture. Listed below are some plants which are classified as male or female:

Male Plants

- Mango – *Mangifera Indica*
- Mauha – *Madhuca Indica*
- Teak – *Tectona Grandis*
- Amla – *Embelica Officinatis*
- Fig – *Ficus Glomerata*
- Coconut with water – *Cocos nucifera*
- Hirda – *Terminellia Chebulla*
- Banana – *Musa paradisica*
- Drumstick – *Moringa olifera*
- Shid – *Bauhinia racemosa*

Female Plants

- Halad – Turmeric – *Curcuma domestica*
- Kharik – *Phoenix species*
- Papaya – *Carcica Papaya*
- Cotton – *Caltropis gigantean*
- Jamun – *Eugenia jambolina*
- Palas – *Beutea frondosa*

Thus according to the Thakars each plant, animal (including man) has male and female elements in their respective bodies.

(m) Concept of Age/Growth

Plants also go through various stages of growth during their lifetime like the human beings. Plants are green and healthy when young just like youths.

The Worm Attack: Worms and white ants attack plant and more often than not cause decay and disease in plants. The human body is also believed to be attacked by worms (*Kide*) which cause disease. Eg. Scabies is believed to be caused by the *Jantu* (germs) which suck blood (*Raghat*) when it becomes sweet. Therefore to neutralise this sweetness bitter plants are taken as medicines. Thus scabies is perceived as an internal rather an external disorder and the Thakars therefore mock at the PHC doctors who advice them to use soap on the infected parts.

Manure Vs Food: The plants obtain nutrition from the manure like compost, farm yard manure. This manure helps plants grow. In a similar way the human body obtains nourishment from food. Lack of manure and food in the plants and humans respectively leads to weakness which at times is fatal.

Survival: The survival of the human body, plant body and *atma* depends on a continuous proportionate supply of water, sunlight/moonlight, air, fire or heat (*Agni*) and food.

The above mentioned elements have their sources in:

1. Sun, Moon (Male Gods) – light;
2. Wind (Female God) – wind;
3. Sun (Male God) – fire;
4. Water (Male God) –water; and
5. Natural environment – food.

The morphology of human body is made up of mud (mother Earth-female). Plants have profoundly influenced the culture and civilisation of man (Choudhari 1981). Traditional tales, mythological stories, events in epics, religious worships, and festivals, rituals of births, puberty, marriage and death, in many cultures have references to plant symbols and their meanings in human social system.

Plants have been the oldest associates of man and therefore form an integral part of human culture. The fact that plants have found usage in rituals and ceremonies proves that they have symbolic and meaningful values.

An attempt is made to highlight the plant symbols in the Thakar culture and their association with the human body.

To demonstrate the manner in which the Thakar's interpret human body as a part of the universe and nature (i.e. plants).

(i) Butea Frondosa (*Palas*) Family: Papilionaceae

This plant is classified by the Thakars as belonging to the feminine gender. It is used in many rituals and ceremonies where it symbolizes or is associated with human body.

BIRTH CONTROL RITUAL

Soon after birth of a child, the midwife (*Suine*) cuts and buries the umbilical chord (*nal*) and the placental waste (*var*) as a preventive measure, so that the cord and the waste may not become an object of sorcery and witchcraft.

The midwife takes a *palas* leaf, places on it the umbilical chord in the centre with some rice, *gulal* (red powder), a coin and a wick. The leaf is then buried (along with the things placed on it) on the outside of the western wall of the house. A temporary bathing place is made for the mother and the child to bathe. Thus the used bath water is allowed to flow over the buried *palas* leaf as the water helps the chord to decay and perish.

Meanings

- The *Palas* leaf – symbolises the woman.
- Leaf placed with its dorsal side upwards – this symbolises the sexual position of the fertile woman.
- Apex of the Leaf – symbolises the woman's head.
- Central part of the leaf – is symbolic of the womb.
- *Var* (Placental waste) – placed in the central part of the leaf is symbolic of the uterus in which the child is nurtured.
- Umbilical Chord – Symbolises the child.
- Gulal (red powder) – symbolises the menstrual blood of the woman, her fertility.
- Rice – the rice is symbolic of the continuity of fertility.
- Wick (*Wat*) – symbolises the presence of the Sun (masculine nature). It is believed that the light of the Sun and fire help the *atma* (soul) of the mother and child to survive.
- East-west placement of the leaf—is symbolic of two aspects:
    - Delivery posture of the woman.
    - Sexual posture of the woman.
- The base of the petioie – symbolises the vaginal opening. The dorsal placing of the leaf signifies the woman's desire for having more children.

The Turning Over of the Palas Leaf

Chaphekar L.N.(1960:45) states that a Thakar woman who does not wish to bar anymore children buries the placenta of the child in an inverted position. The meaning of this action according to the Thakar midwives and elderly woman meant the concerned family must put an end to producing more children. The symbolic elements associated with this action are related to social control designed culturally through spiritual media i.e. *'Satvai'* (mother Earth's desire or wish for the family to stop producing children).

This ritual expresses or symbolizes a cultural check on population growth.

The Cosmic Elements Associated with the Burial Rite of the Umbilical Chord

The fertility of a woman, her sexual behaviour, her feminine nature etc., is on the whole linked to mother earth by the Thakars. They believe that the dorsal side of the mother Earth faces the Sun – her husband and all life on earth are their offspring.

At the time of the burial (of the *palas* leaf) a wick is placed on the *palas* leaf. The wick is symbolic of the Sun's posture during sex with the mother Earth. The water which flows on the buried leaf symbolises the flow of spermatic fluid of the Sun into the mother Earth. This sexual union of the Sun and the Earth at cosmic level is prevalent in the Thakar culture.

Marriage Ritual and *Palas* Leaf

The *palas* leaf is also used in the wedding rituals by the Thakars. During the wedding, the bride is separated from the groom by a curtain, while the Brahman (priest) chants the scriptures.

The bride places her left foot on the *palas* leaf and the groom places his right foot on another *palas* and apex of the two leaves point towards the east in case of bridegroom and west in case of the bride. As soon as the chanting of scriptures is completed, the curtain falls.

The falling of the curtain symbolises the union of these two leaves, thereby uniting symbolically two physical bodies into a social unit (family). The overlapping of the male (bridegroom's) leaf over the female (bride's) leaf symbolises the social sanction given by the Thakar society for these two to have sexual relationship, to be fertile and fruitful.

NATURE AND ROLE OF ETHNO-MEDICAL SPECIALISTS

As any highly developed society tends to have its specialised personnel, so does the folk society. If help is sought from medical practitioners, various types of specialists may be available, including herbalists, shamans, midwives, bonesetters and masseurs. A therapist may specialise in only one type of skill or may combine several in the practice, while there is considerable material on distinction among the traditional therapists based on the variation in specialisation (Nurge 1958: Lieban 1962, Maclean 1969). The qualitative data collected on the practitioners of Thakars has revealed that there are 7 types of medical practitioners rendering health care services to their fellowmen since time immemorial. Each one has got a special role in treating and taking care of the sick in their community. These practitioners are as follows:

1. *Bhagat* : A male socio-ritual curer
2. *Bhagatin* : A female socio-ritual curer
3. *Vaidu* : Herbalist
4. *Had Vaidu* : Bone setter
5. *Mantrik* : A specialised Herbalist expert in Scorpion stings and Snake bites
6. *Suine* : Mid-wife
7. *Potdhari* : Assistant mid-wife.

1. *Bhagat*

A *Bhagat* is the principle medical specialist among all the other Thakar specialists. He is a professional socio-ritual curer, a diviner and an interpreter of supernatural phenomenon. A *Bhagat* is one who is proficient in *bhakti*, which is a meaningful art of establishing contact with the supernatural beings and hence carried out by a *Bhagat* because he is culturally assigned to serve his society members.

As stated by Sudhir Kakar (1982:89), that *Bhagat* may be compared to *Shamans* who generally specialise in script illness and generally salient characteristic of a *Shamans* is in their ability to go into voluntary and controlled trance, during their diagnostic or healing efforts.

A Thakar on the other hand describes the diagnostic rites and process of trance during the healing rites as a meaningful situation or event. They believe this action to be symbolic of entry of divine power into the *Bhagat's* body which helps him to judge the origin and cause of illness. A *Bhagat* gets power to diagnose and heal from "Sun" – the creator of universe and life.

It is very necessary for a *Bhagat* to continue to cure unless he gets a vision from the Sun God to give up his profession. If he stops, he is suspected to have devoted himself to sorcery. He must also practice his profession to fulfill his religious duty assigned to him by "Sun God". He does not work for money. A famous *Bhagat* may pay a visit to another village, if called upon. A *Bhagat* is always respected and given a higher status by the members of his society as an image of high moral and ethics. He is a mediator between God and his society. A *Bhagat* plays dual roles as farmer and as a medical practitioner for his society. The office of a *Bhagat* is socially transmitted from one generation to other in a family.

2. *Bhagatin*

A *Bhagatin* is a female *Shaman*. She holds the same status in her society as the *Bhagat* goes. A *Bhagatin* gets the power of healing and diagnosing the cause of an illness from "*Dantari*" (Mother Earth) and the "*Baya*" (Planetary spirits/sisters of Mother of Earth). Her method of diagnosis also differs from the *Bhagat*. She gets into a trance "*Angat Vara Yeto*" while the *Bhagat* uses the metal pot technique.

A *Bhagatin* has destructive powers; she can cast magico-religious spells on her enemies, whereas a *Bhagat* has protective powers and therefore he is superior and a more capable practitioner than a *Bhagatin*. A *Bhagatin* also has some knowledge of herbal medicine and prescribes it for mostly health problems of woman. She cures both male and female patients, while female patients prefer to go her first, in case she is not able to cure then they consult the *Bhagat*.

Medical Functions of *Bhagats* and *Bhagatins*

The medical functions of a *Bhagat* and *Bhagatin* are broadly classified by them are as follows:

Diagnosis of the Origin and Cause of Illness

Shamanism is related to a system of beliefs about the causes and cures of diseases, within a given cultural frame of reference. The healing performance of a *Shaman* takes place in a group context, and the drama of diagnosing and healing is given a public recognition. The patient is surrounded by familiar people in a ceremonial or ritualistic situation to which he has become accustomed through witnessing curing rites for others.

Diagnosis of illness begins after setting the necessary objects of worship, cleaning rites of *Bhagats* and *Bhagatins*, chanting prayers to "Sun" – in the case of *Bhagat* and "Mother Earth" – in the case of *Bhagatin*, laying the offering, music instruments (in this case drum – *Dholki*). The action of setting a stage of healing to start the diagnosis rite symbolically draws into operation on objective reality, by giving that situation or context a culturally recognised meaning.

The Diagnosis Rite

The methods, techniques or rituals of diagnosing illness differ from community to community. Among the Bhils of Dhule district, in the State of Maharashtra the *Shaman* (Badwa) uses prayer beads (*abrus precatorius*) to diagnose the origin and cause of illness. While the Koknas of Jawhar, Thane district use rice grains which are spread in a shifter to diagnose illness. (Tibhuwan Robin 188: 58).

There are two types of diagnostic rituals performed separately by the *Bhagat* and the *Bhagatin* to diagnose the cause of illness of their patients.

1. The metal pot technique (*Tambya phirawane*)
2. Getting into trance (*Vara yene*).

The metal pot technique (*Tambya phirawane*) is used by a *Bhagat*, while the *Bhagatin* gets into trance to trace the origin and cause of illness. The *Bhagat* also gets into trance at times to diagnose the cause of illness. Regarding what these two techniques are, how they are ritually performed, what objects are used and what 'ill' means to the Thakars are highlighted in detail in the case studies of *Bhagats* and *Bhagatins* in this chapter. Thus, diagnosis is one of the most important aspect of the medical functions of a *Bhagat* and a *Bhagatin*.

Interpretations of the origin and cause of illness is followed by the diagnosis ritual. The diagnosis techniques help the *Bhagats* and *Bhagatins* to trace the cause. Interpretation of the cause of illness is done on the basis of following pathogenic agents which can bring about illness.

Pathogenic Agents/Forces

1.	*Phirta Mela*	: The moving Planetary Spirits.
2.	*Zokyachya Devi*	: The Goddesses of Swing who dwell on the mountains.
3.	*Chokhy/Ratya Baya*	: The Spirits (Female) of the Devjati (upper caste)
4.	*Gandhicha Tap*	: Measles (Baya)
5.	*Kilyachya Devi*	: Goddesses of the Fort
6.	*Germany Baya*	: Spirits of the Britishers
7.	*Fodya Baya*	: Goddess of Smallpox
8.	*Vanachi Baju*	: Evil force of the forest
9.	*Pisha, Munja & Khais*	: Male Evil Spirits
10.	*Hadeli*	: Female Evil Spirits
11.	*Satvai*	: Mother Earth
12.	*Ilkat Mal Bhut*	: Evil Spirit of Wealth
13.	*Shel Bhut*	: Spirit of the goats
14.	*Kolha Bhut*	: Evil Spirit of the Fox
15.	*Waghya, Chedha, Khambya, Bhairi*	: Village Gods
16.	*Mariai*	: Goddess of the Mahar Caste

(Contd...)

17.	*Bhavani*	: Goddess of the Mahar Caste
18.	*Malavarcha Chedha*	: The God of the Loft
19.	*Panch Mukhee Chedha*	: The five hooded Cobra
20.	*Gupit Bhut*	: Secret Evil Spirit
21.	*Dith Bhut*	: Spirit of the Evil Eye
22.	*Mari Bhut*	: Evil Spirit of the Mahar Caste
23.	*Vir / Supali*	: Ancestral Spirits
24.	*Kuldev*	: Clan Gods.

The above mentioned pathogenic agents are believed to cause illness. Depending on the cultural situations or context in which the illness might have occurred, the *Bhagat* or *Bhagatin* interpret one of the pathogenic agents responsible for causing illness.

Disease Treatment

The second most important function of a *Bhagat* and *Bhagatin* is treatment of disease using magico-religious and ritualistic healing techniques. There are again three types of treatments given by the *Shamans*:

1. *Herbal Therapy:* This is purely administration of medicinal herbs or medical extracts of animals in a ritualistic fashion.
2. *Magico-ritualistic treatment:* This involves the diagnosis rites, healing rites, the rites of offering coconuts, sacrifices, rituals of pleasing the pathogenic agents, driving out evil spirits, neutralising evil effect and so on.
3. *Combination of magico-ritualistic and Herbal / chemotherapy:* This involves both medication as well as ritualistic performance so as to give physical and psychological relief to the patient.

Medical Advice

One of the most important jobs of the *Bhagats* and *Bhagatins* is to render free medical advice to their patients on the following aspects:

- The pathogenic agents that cause disease and the situation in which the diseases are caused.
- How to prevent these pathogenic agents from causing illness.
- Advice on dangerous areas such as, where the evil spirit, the Rakshas (Giants) and other pathogenic agents dwell.
- The care that people must take and observe taboos of health.
- Advice on maintaining good relationship with the pathogenic agents.
- Advice on keeping certain holy objects or charmed objects to prevent illness.
- Performing and presiding over healing rituals.
- Offering coconuts and sacrifices and so on

3. *Vaidu*

A *Vaidu* (Herbalist) is one who has a vast knowledge of Herbal medicines and heals his patients only by giving herbal therapy. He prepares medicines from various plant parts such as root, shoot, bark, leaf, flower, seed, fruit etc. Besides administering medicinal herbs he also uses animal extracts for treating his patients. He also advises his patients on diet.

It was observed that although a *Vaidu* deals with only Chemotherapy there is a lot of ritualistic behaviour associated with his profession which is common to that of a *Bhagat*. This ritualistic behaviour associated with collections, preparation and administration of medicines, the social taboos of his professions, the religious elements associated with his profession are all described in the case study form in this chapter.

4. *Had Vaidu*

A Had Vaidu (Bone Setter) is one who has a sound knowledge of the location of various nerves, veins and bones in the human body. He heals fractures, swellings, sprains, joint pains etc using various herbal medicines.

He is an expert masseur, a bone setter and a skilled brandsman. As a masseur he uses various medicated oils such as Mauha Seed Oil (*Bacia latifolia*); Karanj Seed Oil (*Pongamia pinnata*); Mutton and Chicken fat oil and of course groundnut oil. He is a master bone setter among the Thakar medical practitioners. Branding is another form of therapy used by him. He heats iron rod and gently touches it on painful parts of the body. The branding technique is popularly known as '*Chocha Dena*'. Other details of Thakars bone setters are presented in a case study form in this chapter.

5. *Mantrik*

A *Mantrik* is a specialised herbalist, who deals specifically with healing scorpion stings and snakebites, using *Mantra* techniques. He has a vast knowledge about the behaviour of different species of snakes and scorpions and hence gives herbal cure to his patients, of course ritually accompanied by his *Mantras* which he chants to give his patient psychological relief initially.

Mantrik's office in a Thakar society is hereditary i.e. it is passed on from generation to generation. He undergoes a lengthy period of training and apprenticeship under the leadership and guidance of his Guru.

During his early phase of learning *Mantras*, a *Mantrik* is expected to get into the river right in the middle on a '*Poornima*' (full moon night) or '*Amosha*' (no moon night) to learn his *Mantras*. He takes 50 stones with him each time he recites his *Mantras* he will throw a stone in the water. This he does for 50 times. He is expected to be totally naked while he is in water. This is a sought of assignment for him which he does for a year or so especially during summer and winter season for every fortnight.

Mantrik is so deeply specialised in curing snakebites and scorpion stings that he can handle almost any patient, however seriously he may be bitten.

Maruti Dalu Ughda a famous *Mantrik* of Sarai Wadi (hamlet) is known for curing scorpion and snakebitten patients.

My informant Ramchandra Lobhie said, Maruti makes his patients face towards east. If the patient is bitten by a poisonous snake Dalu jumps in the well with a tumbler and goes right at the bottom of the well and get water from there. He splashes this water on his patients face five times very hard. Then gives a herbal cure, while he is splashing water he chants *Mantras* taking the name of God Bhairi who is the source of healing power to a *Mantrik*.This act in most cases take away the fear of the patient even if he is not bitten by a poisonous snake.

Maruti was quite expert in curing his patients that he can exactly trace the snake which bit his patient, from the marks of the teeth.

A *Mantrik* also knows a lot of preventive remedies for cultural etiologies as well as other natural causes of illness.

6. *Suine (Midwife)*

In almost all the Thakar hamlets deliveries take place at home, because of the cultural and ritualistic importance of the child birth ceremonies, which are carried out by *Suine* (a birth attendant).

The duties of a *Suine* are to give advice and medical aid to the expectant mother, to assist in delivering the baby and to treat any illnesses that might befall the new mother and infant. She has a vast knowledge of child birth techniques also the cultural behaviour expected during pregnancy and childbirth. She is also a masseur and knows the proper diet for the mother and child.

Although her knowledge of herbal medicine is not that extensive like the *Vaidus* and *Bhagats*, she does know some medicinal plants for ailments like urinary disorders, abortions etc. Bhagubai Darwade a *Suine* of Bor Wadi knows a number of medicines and hence is a popular *Suine* of Kikwi village.

To become a *Suine* woman starts watching an accomplished *Suine* go about her duties. The office of a *Suine* is not exactly hereditary, but in most cases mothers tend to teach their daughters the skills of child birth. Most *Suines* teach their daughters-in-law the art of attending to a child birth and delivery.

A *Suine* always sees that a delivering mother faces the 'East' (a direction always associated with life). If a child is stillborn, mother's face is immediately turned to South (a direction always perceived by the Thakars and associated with death). Placental waste (*var*) and the umbilical chord (*nal*) is buried on the western part of the house just adjacent to the cowdung plastered wall outside. A hole about 1foot is dug to bury the umbilical chord to prevent it from being a tool of witchcraft.

At the same time the child and the mother bathe inside the house just opposite to the place of umbilical chord, for five days. A *Suine* gives bath to the child for twelve days. On the fifth day, which is a very important day because it is on this day the child's fortune is written by *Satvai* (Goddess of fortune) who comes in the form of a bird, cat, rat, dog, cow, etc. to visit the child.

On the fifth day at 8 o'clock in the evening the bathing place is worshipped, indirectly the *Satvai* is worshipped and food is kept for her to eat. This ceremony is headed by the *Suine*.

A *Suine* plays an important role in taking decisions, especially when it comes to repeated abortions and still births, which are attributed to sexual intercourse with evil spirits namely *Khais* and *Munja*. Congenital deformities etc. are also attributed to breach of pregnancy taboos.

A severely deformed child is killed and buried, since he is believed to be a product of evil spirit and would be dangerous to the Thakar community. This decision of identifying the child as product of *Khais* or *Munja* is certainly taken by the *Suine*.

On the 12th day after a child is born it is put in the traditional swing (*Jholi*) and it is on this day the *Suine* is awarded a gift depending on the financial capacity of the donor. Mostly she gets a blouse piece, bangles and 5-10 rupees for the 12 days of service which she has rendered to the child and the mother.

7. *Potdhari (Assistant Midwife)*

The very word *potdhari* means a helper who holds the stomach or an assistant midwife. A *potdhari* helps the *Suine* in delivering a child. Any midwife practices as a *potdhari* for 4-5 years till she becomes a perfectly trained mid-wife.

In case of emergency, that when a midwife is not available in the village, the *potdhari* performs the delivery. She has a little knowledge of home remedies for minor ailments or helath problems that befall the new child and mother. A *potdhari* gets 3-10 rupees for her services rendered in delivering a child, depending on the socio-economic status of the family which the child is born. About other details of a *potdhari*, see case study in this chapter.

DISCUSSION

It is important to note that despite of 57 years of independence, the rapid influence of modernisation and urbanisation the tribals of India still cling on to their traditional beliefs and practices of body image, human reproduction and birth control. On the other hand we have a vast network of primary health care service system and health care and education provides, who have allopathic background and consider the tribal beliefs and practices as superstitious. There is a need to give a serious thought to this issue.

5

Ethno-medical Therapies for Contraception and Impotency Among Santhals

PROFILE OF SANTHALS

Origin/History

The Santhals are the third largest tribal community of India, with a population of more than 5 million. They are distributed across the states of Bihar, West Bengal, Orissa and Tripura. The Santhals are a well studied community for more than a century. They are unique in many ways. They even use a script invented just 80 years ago. The *Olchiki* script was an epoch-making invention, which provided appropriate writing symbols to the Santhals.

Quintessentially, the Santhals locate their lifestyle and worldview in cooperation, mutual care and love. Their cultural expressions in nature, sound, language, creativity and sensitivity treat all life forms as sacred and respect them for what they are. Not only forms of life but even inanimate things and phenomena of nature are regarded as sacred. The sacredness is re-established in metaphors, rituals, songs, dance and everyday practices. This is the pristine, primal vision from which the new world order has much to learn. At home, they speak the Santhali language, but with outsiders they can communicate in Hindi or in Bengali, depending upon the region.

In contrast to the strife of the class and caste ridden societies of today, the following are the main socio-religious characteristics of the Santhals:

The society is devoid of caste hierarchy. The Santhal's is a casteless society; By birth no person, family, clan group is superior or inferior; Image or idol worship is absent and there is no temple in Santhal society; Blood offering is prevalent in the community; Earlier practice of cow sacrifice is now restricted; Both burial and cremation are practiced. A chicken is dedicated to the dead body; Offering during worship is made within the pictorial boundary known as *khond* as a mark of the mundane relationship of the supernatural power; Priesthood is not appropriated by a particular clan group or a sect but is owned by the family members of the first settlers of the village. Occasionally selection of a successor of the old priest is held if he leaves no issue (male child). Such a selection is made mainly by a divinated person and it is undisputed.

Traditional Beliefs

One idea which gets repeated in traditional thought and culture is the inseparability of nature and culture. There is an implicit acceptance of the fact that human beings constitute an integral part of nature. This is most explicit among indigenous communities such as the Santhals, which thrive in the lap of nature. The ritual language paves the way of life. The Santhals live with nature of which they are an inseparable part. The Santhals have understood the basic relatedness of nature and culture, without the imposition of a theory based on creation or evolution. Briefly, the traditional Santhal culture is the prime extant example of a lifestyle that has proved its capacity to integrate with the natural and the supernatural world.

The association between tribal life and animals is very strong because they have lived together from the ancient times. The Santhal knowledge about the origin of animals on the earth is in line with the present day scientific opinion and they have vast experience of the use of animals for various requirements at every level.

Santhals believe that food is for energy and it also saves life, and it is made of Solid, Liquid and Gas. In accordance to their theory, our body is like a machine and food is similar to oil necessary for it and they also believe that the kind of food one takes makes a great impact on body.

The Santhals have their own and well defined conception of sound. Sounds are always an important indicator of anything going on inside or outside the village; certain sounds are attributed to auspiciousness or inauspiciousness. The voices of humans, animals and nature blend into a harmonious, constantly moving stream of sound. It is observed that some sounds are auspicious or inauspicious in relation to variables like time, space, direction and object. In spite of the 'auspicious, and the inauspicious', as observed by Saraswati, they are transcendental categories, each accommodating within itself a great amount of variations and uses.

The Santhals have been preserving similarity between sound and symbol. The very ingenuity in shaping the symbols and arrangement of the script has been greatly helpful in transmission of the script. A large number of words in the language of Santhals derive from natural sounds. This is illustrated in the paper of Khageswar Mahapatra complemented with Shyam Sunder Mohapatra's essay, which explains that the words in *Ol Chiki* are derived from the physical environment and what surrounds the people—hills, rivers, trees, birds, bees, plough, sickle—the list is endless.

The Santhals believe that there are gods everywhere. They worship the *Bonga buru*. The worldview is conditioned by the socio-cultural situation of a community. The Santhal worldview incorporates Man, Nature and God and the relationship that exists between these components. The Santhal's situate their lifestyle and worldview in cooperation, mutual care and love. There are many such rituals and festivals observed by the Santhals.

In Santhal opinion, agricultural land is the most valuable resource as it is everlasting and does not change like the material items. And they have very close ties with nature, which surrounds the human society. They believe in supernatural beings and their ancestral spirits also. The Santhals are fully aware of their position in group commonality.

The Santhali language is part of the Austro-Asiatic family, distantly related to Vietnamese and Khmer. The Santhali script, or *Ol Chiki*, is alphabetic, and does not share any of the syllabic properties of the other Indic scripts such as Devanagari. It uses 30 letters and five basic diacritics. It has 6 basic vowels and three additional vowels, generated using the *Gahla Tudag*.

The Santhal people love music and dance. Like other Indian people groups, their culture has been influenced by mainstream Indian culture and by Western culture, but traditional music and dance still remain. They believe in supernatural beings and ancestral spirits. The Santhal system of governance, known as *Manjhi–Paragana*, may be compared to what is often called Local Self Governance. This body is responsible for making decisions to ameliorate the village's socio-economic condition.

The Santhals live in patriarchal communities with village based governance structures. A village headman, *Manjhi*, is supported by other village officers including a *Paranik* (deputy), *Godet* (assistant), *Naike* (religious leader) and *Jog Manjhi* (upholder of morals of the youth). These officers oversee ceremonies, give guidance and support to villagers and administer the Santhal laws on trespass, marriage, divorce, theft etc. There is a three tier structure of customary courts beginning with the village court (a gathering of all male head of households, presided over by the *Manjhi*), the *more hor* (meeting of five *Manjhi's* of the area, presided over by a *Parganait*), and the *lo bir* (traditionally held during the annual hunt and comprising all male heads of households of a large number of villages). In each court the outcome is said to be a collective decision of all those present – the *Manjhi* or *Parganait* listens to the discussion and summarises the major consensus by way of conclusion. Outcomes generally aim to correct the wrong that has occurred through compensation or to punish the perpetrator with a fine (this may be a meal or drink given to those present at the gathering).

Santhal law governs not only disputes, but also important social aspects of life – marriage, birth, death, illness. Adherence to the law is not simply a matter of avoiding punishment; it is a sign of commitment to the village community and to the hierarchy of the village officers and elders.

The Santhals have a special spring festival of rejoicing with sprinkling of water, special songs and dances. When the roles of the deities are acted out by men, and thereby many traditional social barriers fall. Usually, the supreme God is not offered any specific worship among tribals. But among the Santhals of Mayurbhanj, one may perform the worship every fifth year or at least one in a life-time. Bondo festivities have a great relevance for the tribal communities of Orissa. The Bondos spend a great deal of time on their religion, and the feasts and holidays are an important part of Bondo life. Moreover, the collective festivities foster a sense of solidarity of the village and fortify one's confidence in undertaking major activities in economic and social life as possible. Thus, she proves herself to be virtuous and devoted. The wife presents a number of delicacies to her husband at the end of her fast.

Pusha Punein is celebrated by the tribesmen of north Orissa, specially the Bhuiyan, the Gond and others. They celebrate this festival on a day closet to the actual full moon day of month. The whole village joins in the celebrations of feasting, drinking and dancing.

Role in the Freedom Struggle: Santhal Rebellion

On 30 June 1855, two Santhal rebel leaders, Sidhu and Kanhu Murmu, mobilised ten thousand Santhals and declared a rebellion against British colonists. The Santhals initially gained some success but soon the British found out a new way to tackle these rebels. As the legend goes that the Santhals so skilled in archery could throw arrows extremely accurate and with great power.The British soon understood that there was no point fighting them in the forest but to force them come out of the forest. So in a conclusive battle which followed the British equipped with modern firearms and war elephants stationed themselves at the foot of the hill.When the battle began the British officer ordered fire without bullet as the Santhals could not trace this trap set by the much experienced [British] war strategy charged with full potential. This step proved to be disastrous for them since as soon as they neared the foot of the hill the British army attacked with full power and this time using bullet. Thereafter attacking every village of the Santhals and making sure that the last drop of revolutionary spirit was annihilated. Although the revolution was brutally suppressed, it marked a great change in the colonial rule and policy. The day is still celebrated among the Santhal community with great respect and spirit for the thousands of the Santhal martyrs who sacrificed their lives along with their two celebrated leaders to win freedom from the rule of the Jamindars and the British operatives.

Geographical Distribution

Before the advents of the British in India Santhals resided peacefully in the hilly districts of Cuttack, Dhalbhum, Manbhum, Barabhum, Chhotanagpur, Palamau, Hazaribagh, Midnapur, Bankura and Birbhum.They started their agrarian way of life by clearing the forest and also engaged themselves in hunting for subsistence.

Sub-tribes

The Santhals call themselves *Hor*, which means man. The community is divided into two groups, namely Deswali Santhal and Kharwar Santhal. The Kharwar are the followers of a reformist cult. The largest contribution of Santhals in Bihar, and a large corpus of literature in Bengali as well as in Santhali exist that fictionalises Santhal life and culture. In Bihar, the Santhals are also known as Manjhi. The Santhals believe that they originated from Pilchu Haram and Pilchu Burhi, and their legends describe prolonged wandering before they reached their present habitat. This is resonant with historical experience, since traditionally the Santhals were resident of the Chhota Nagpur Plateau, and after the famine of 1770 came to Birbhum and Santhal Paragana.

Clans

A total 12 clans are found among the Santhals. They are *Hansdak', Murmu, Hembrom, Soren, Kisku, Tudu, Marndi, Baske, Besra, Chonre, Puria and Bedea*. An affiliation or sacred contact is believed to link these clans and their respective totems. Therefore, each of the names of clans is derived from either from the plants or animals species. There is a belief that is prevalent among the Santhals that totems have some connection with the deeds or birth of ancestors of the clans. *Hansdak'* clan members claim to be of the highest status as they have derived from the name of their clan from first ancestors. The term *Hans* designates wild goose while *dak'* in Santhali means water. This clan is, therefore, linked to the original state of world and first ancestors. It is the most senior among the all clans of the Santhals since it is related to myth of creation. Moreover, swan or goose is not just animal. It builds nest on earth, walks on earth and flies on sky.

Physical Features

A few of the Indian anthropologists also believe that humans first came to India about 65000-55000 years ago. The earliest of them were Proto-Australoids followed by the Proto-Dravidians. The Proto-Australoids can be identified with some facial characteristics such as low forehead, thick lips, wide jaw and wavy hair. Historians believe that they were the ancestors of the tribal community residing in the eastern part of India (excluding hilly portions). So the Santhals, Kols and Mundas may be the descendants of them.

Family Type

Within the Santhal village each household has a duty to foster this sense of community. However, despite this, the household unit remains largely autonomous of the community. Privacy is respected and the village will not intervene in a household dispute unless they are called to intervene by a family member. The household has its own structure and codes of behaviour, which are semi-autonomous of the village legal order.

Use of alcoholic drink is very common among them. Rice-beer is their traditional drink which is extensively used on the occasion of festivals and socio-religious ceremonies. They prepare this drink at home and purchase Mahua liquor from the local vendors.

They observe Karama festival and Makar Sankranti elaborately. Celebration of socio-religious ceremonies like birth, marriage and death are marked by dancing, singing and drinking. The Santhals work as cultivators and agricultural labourers. After the agricultural season is over they generally migrate for a temporary period to work as daily wagers.

Marriage

According to the Santhals, the world is divided into *Hor* and *Diku*, or the Santhal and the Non Santhals. Spouses can be acquired through negotiation, elopement and capture, though negotiation is preferred. A married Santhal woman puts vermilion in the parting of her hair. There is a custom of bride price among the Santhals, but recently dowry has become common among the well-to-do Santhals. Age at marriage normally is 15-18 for girls, and 16-22 years for boys. After marriage, the bride lives at the husband's home, and divorce is permitted with the permission of the village council.

The marriage negotiations are done by match makers called *Bartul* and *Raibareik*. The bride is selected in consultation with her father and close relatives. Payment of bride price is called *Gonong* among Santhals.

Birth Rituals/Ceremonies

Among the Santhals the father is not allowed to enter the house when the baby is getting delivered. The period of birth pollution is followed as well, it is 3 days in case a girl is born and 5 days if the baby is male child, after this period, purificatory bath is taken by the entire family. The purificatory bath and the ceremony attached to it are called "*Janam Chattihar*". The male members shave their heads and beard and at last shave the head of the child, and then they go the nearest pond to take bath. The midwife ties a thread soaked in turmeric around the child's waist. Then the child and the members of the family and the village are purified with rice flour and water. Later the child is given the name by its parents and declared in front of the village, which generally corresponds with the name of any of the dead relative. The ceremony ends with a drink called – *Neem Dak Mandi*.

Puberty Rituals/Ceremonies

The boys and girls on attaining puberty must perform – *Chacho Chattihar* – in order to be admitted as the full-fledged member in the society. This allows them to attend the communal worship of the deities in the village and eat sacrificial meat. The ceremony is performed by serving rice beer to the assembled villagers, followed by dancing and singing. This ceremony has to be performed before the marriage or death of that person; otherwise it is considered that the impurities of the youth are not washed off.

Death Rituals

Participation of the community members is more at the time of death than at the time of birth ceremonies. As soon as the person dies, the near kins and relatives rush to the house of bereaved family. No formal invitation is extended to kinsmen, however, the whole village joins the funeral procession, the dead are buried and the village members cover the grave by putting handful of earth in the grave. With the death of the person the village gets polluted and worship of the village deity is prohibited till first *bhoj* is observed.

Soul Migration Rituals

The Santhals believe in the presence of the souls of their dead whom they worship. The village deities like *Marang Baru*, literally the mountain spirits figure prominently in most of their mythological folklores, because he is supposed to be sharing the fortunes of the village and protects the villagers from evil things. Deities of diseases like small pox and abortion are considered as evil spirits and cause of death is considered to be the bad effect of evil spirits.

About the Santhals of Malda district in West Bengal, A.B. Chaudhuri, an officer of the Indian Police Service, wrote in his book *Witch Killings Amongst Santhals* (Ashish Publishing House, New Delhi; 1984; Rs.150) that faced with a desolate existence and haunted by extreme poverty and helplessness, the tribe had started to look to Mahans for leadership. *Mahan* is "one who knows", and is assisted by kavirajs. He is supposed to know tribal lore and be able to unravel the mysteries of time. A witch is called the *fuskin* here, and whenever there is a drought or a famine or a disease, the tribal people run to the *Mahan*, who would identify some hapless woman as the *fuskin*. In almost all cases of witch-killing, Chaudhuri noted that the aged and the weak were identified as witches. The tribal people do not consider it a sin to kill a *fuskin*. Denying responsibility ends in tragedy, and the *Mahan*'s word is always final. Many a time the poverty-stricken family of the "witch" can only succumb to his decision.

Summoning the denounced woman to the village meeting and assaulting her is a common practice, Chaudhuri noted. Even sons are known to have killed their mothers. The murder of a witch is always preceded by deaths or instances of prolonged illness in the village or family. Often sickness and land disputes coincided so perfectly that it was difficult to discern which the real reason was for a woman having been declared a *fuskin*. Chaudhuri argues in his book that the distrust in women has been accentuated by a belief that they are superior to men in matters of *mantras* or incantations. Should they be allowed to worship the *Bongas*, (the supreme deities) they would win favour quickly and their nature being destructive, they would invariably indulge in destructive activities to the detriment of society, so went the argument.

It is most likely that cases of witch-killing and persecution of women will continue as long as economic inequities and neglect of the health care infrastructure continue. The reluctance on the part of both the community and the law-enforcers to see the killings of these hapless women as blatant murder, points to collusion among various elements to keep women at the lowest rung of society. To see it merely as a tribal custom would be to ignore the various influences on tribal life, including the political one, where the constitutional right of political participation has the potential to bring women into public life. Revivalism and resistance are but inevitable fallouts.

Religion

According to the Santhal religion, the supreme deity, who ultimately controls the entire universe, is Thakurji. The weight of belief, however, falls on a court of spirits (*bonga*), who handle different aspects of the world and who must be placated with prayers and offerings in order to ward off evil influences. These spirits operate at the village, household, ancestor, and subclan level, along with evil spirits that cause disease, and can inhabit village boundaries, mountains, water, tigers, and the forest. A characteristic feature of the Santhal village is a sacred grove on the edge of the settlement where many spirits live and where a series of annual festivals take place.

The most important spirit is *Maran Buru* (Great Mountain), who is invoked whenever offerings are made and who instructed the first Santhals in sex and brewing of rice beer. *Maran Buru's* consort is the benevolent *Jaher Era* (Lady of the Grove).

A yearly round of rituals connected with the agricultural cycle, along with life-cycle rituals for birth, marriage and burial at death, involves petitions to the spirits and offerings that include the sacrifice of animals, usually birds. Religious leaders are male specialists in medical cures who practice divination and witchcraft. Similar beliefs are common among other tribes of northeast and central India such as the Kharia, Munda, and Oraon. Smaller and more isolated tribes often demonstrate less articulated classification systems of the spiritual hierarchy, described as animism or a generalised worship of spiritual energies connected with locations, activities, and social groups. Religious concepts are intricately entwined with ideas about nature and interaction with local ecological systems. As in Santhal religion, religious specialists are drawn from the village or family and serve a wide range of spiritual functions that focus on placating potentially dangerous spirits and coordinating rituals.

The goddess of small-pox, chicken-pox, cholera, measles and plague epidemics know variously in various regions. They have to be worshipped and offered a sweet drink called '*pana*' at the function of roads leading away from the village. The goddess is asked to leave the supplicant village and save it from their wrath. Among tribals the village deities and some locally believed in Hindu deities are worshipped in some cases with blood sacrifice. Some rites of rain making in drought affected areas are also worshipped by the people of Orissa. Lord Mahadeva in a most common rite is immersed in water so that there may be flood in the area in place of drought. The Santhal tribe of Mayurbhanj district propitiates *Sima Bongas* with promise of special offerings as demanded through the Shaman or spirit-medium. When rains come the promised offerings are made. The hill Bando also makes sacrifices to lessen the fury of rain.

ETHNO-MEDICAL BELIEFS

The Santhals believe in folk medicine. They have their traditional healers upon whom they have considerable faith and confidence. The Santhals have few common characteristics regarding perception of health and disease. Like many other tribal societies they also attribute a lot of diseases to the wrath of God, mischief of evil sprits and magic of human being. Treatment is based upon the removal of causative factor by appeasing God; controlling evil spirits through counter magic, use of sorcery and of course some herbal preparation. Thus religious practices of the Santhals are closely related to their health care system also. Apart from a host of spirits, the pantheon consists of the following deities or *Bongas,* namely:

1. *Sing bonga*: the sun god, the supreme deity, and worshipped after harvesting and before sowing seeds;
2. *Marang buru*: the mountain god is a community as well as a family deity and a guardian god;
3. *Jahera bonga:* the widely celebrated goddess for protection from diseases, She is village deity *(grama devi)* and while displeased can punish with diseases;

4. *Gossain era*: the associate of *Jahera bonga*;
5. *Moreiko and Turuiko:* the deity of fire and are placed in *Jahera,* a place of worship in forest outside village;
6. *Majhi haram* and *Majhi burhi* are protective deities that stop *bongas* and sprits from doing harm to their people.

Besides these deities listed above they have their family deities like "*Ora bongas*" and the "*Abge bonga*". There are 178 different bongas, which the santhals propitiate by magico religious performances.

Creation Myths of Human Bodies

In some songs the Santhals express their quest to find the origin of the earth and man. As they believe, the earth was created first by the earthworm with the help of the turtle. Later, their first ancestral couple sprang from the eggs of two celestial birds, a goose and gander. Thus, the Santhals do not consider earth and man to be direct creations of God. If the sky and earth stand for God and nature respectively, then man is on the side of nature and hence a product of the earth or nature.

In Santhal thought, a human body is considered to be constituted of three fundamental elements of the universe; air, earth and water. But in Santhal songs, only two of them, i.e., air and earth, are described as essentials of human body. Reference to water is made in metaphorical terms, viz., 'water like the spring of life', etc. Water is again referred to in metaphorical terms like the one mentioned earlier. Moreover, of the other two elements; air and earth, air assumes the greatest importance for a human being to survive and is thought to be located in the chest of the human body.

Most of the aspects regarding creation of human body is elucidated in the songs that deal with the creation and the body element are *don* songs of the marriage. This seems to be natural because the marriage-ritual symbolises union of contraries without which any creation or recreation is impossible. Moreover, marriage is the occasion on which the Santhal song of cosmology is recited. The entire song is meant to put the occasion in a wider, universal context of society and tradition. Marriage as an institution, as he adds further, is referred to the beginning of human creation and the particular occasion of the marriage is sought to be viewed in the larger context of the creation of the world, the dawn of human civilisation, the emergence of the Santhal community and its migration in historical times.

There is a belief among the Santhal society about creation of world. They believe that primitive world was filled with only water and God had the problem in creating the land, where man can live. The land is normally considered opposite to water. He created all amphibian animals that can operate both land and water; therefore, he created seven animals—crab, crocodile, alligator, eel, Pawn, earthworm and tortoise. For creating land, God invited the kings of all these animals to solve help him out. Every one was coming one by one; they all had not got any success. Lastly, earthworm came and succeeded to create land. It is said that the King of earthworm after seven days and seven nights ate the bottom of water and excreted in on the back of tortoise that is swimming at the top. The tortoise anchored himself on the both side firmly and brought up the earth and thus earth was shaped. That is why there is a belief among Santhals that earthquakes are result of movement of tortoise. In other words, when tortoise moves or shakes, earthquakes occur in earth. Santhal myth about the creation of world is substantially different from myth associated with creation of world among the other indigenous peoples of India and in many sense it is unique that it ascribe the creation of earth with the help of amphibian animals, specially the earthworm and tortoise. This is all about the story of creation of earth.

There is another interesting myth about creation of human beings. Again here, this myth is substantially different from the many similar myths that are prevalent among the other peoples. Unlike others, Santhal myth is more associated with natures, animals. Although, Santhal do not strictly believe that they have descended from Animals, however, they assume that there is some connection between animal and human being. It reflects many other Santhal beliefs and myth. According to the myth, God created two heavenly birds—Has and Hasil-out of his hair. Then these two birds started flying in the sky. These bird could survive early state of earth, where all earth was covered with water, as they could mediate the opposite elements heaven and earth. It is believed that they flew below the sun and above the earth thus making the contact between the both worlds. After flying several days, they built the nest on the earth and laid the eggs. They are cosmic eggs, out of which two creatures; human male and human female are born—*Pilchu Haram* and *Pilchu Burhi*. Both these myths creation of world and mankind refer the birds and animal as ancestors. Thus Santhal concept of life begins with animals. Therefore, clans' names are after the name of animals.

Potency/Impotency

With regard to infertility and the impotency, conceptually, they perceive that both, the man and the woman could be impotent, and both may not have seeds inside them. So, in order to diagnose whether one is impotent or not, a urine test with mustard oil is conducted, the mixture of the two is taken in the plate, if oil spreads out evenly, then there is no problem, but if does not spread evenly or is rushing into a particular direction then there is further analysis done to find out more about the problem. Based on the diagnosis, drugs, mixture of minerals and plant powders, seed powders are given to the concerned person.

Delivery

For prolonged labour a tablet is made out of the powdered *methi, kapur, tamba bhasm, and kala jeera* and is given to the pregnant mother, this results into delivery immediately and soon the pain is also brought under control.

After delivery women do not go out for almost 2 months and the child is also taken out only after 21 days. A baby born in the 7th month is considered special and having some kind of supreme powers.

Botanical name of plant used	*Local Name*	*Part used*	*Form used*	*Method of preparation*	*Dosage*
Abrus precatorius	Kaaincha	Fruit	Paste	3nos. of fruits with 5gms. of Kankada root, ground to a paste	Taken orally on empty stomach, once every 7th day of menstrual cycle.
Azadirachta indica	Nimba	Seed	Oil	–	Applied externally as it is spermicidal.
Ferula assafoetida	Hingu	Fruit	Powder	5gm of assafoetida mashed with ripe banana	Taken orally on empty stomach, once every 7th day of menstrual cycle.
Ricinus communis	Jada	Seed	Peeled seed	3nos. of seeds are peeled	-do-
Ocimum sanctum	Tulasi	Leaves	Decoction	40ml of decoction	Taken orally on empty stomach, once daily for 5days from 5th day of menstrual cycle.
Syzygium aromaticum	Labanga	Fruit	-	3 nos. of fruits	Chewed daily after rising in the morning (Before washing mouth)
Piper longum	Long pepper	Fruit	Powder		3 gm daily with luke warm milk at the bed time
Embelia ribes	Bidanga	Fruit			
Borax			Paste	5gm flower with 5gm jaggery	Taken for theree days after menstrual cycle serves for birth control for one month.

Apart from the abovementioned plants, the following plants have said to have ethno-medicinal uses mainly in terms of contraceptives, abortion inducing agents, medicines that ease the delivery process and medicines that ensure secretion of breast milk by Santhals.

Treatment of Umbilical Cord and Breast Feeding

Cutting of the umbilical cord is done by the *Dai*, as per the tradition, nowadays, blade is used. Breast feeding is initiated only after the umbilical cord is cut, in case if she is late and taking too much time then immediately it is done but mostly people wait for the *Dai*. The colostrum milk is given to the newborn, however, if the breast milk is insufficient, then the mother is fed with *Thentai Mulla* – it's a small plant and the juice of the root of this plant is given.

Immediately after the delivery of the baby, in fifteen minutes time; the root of the Oppa Narangi – bark of the Karanji tree is made into a juice given to the mother, the understanding is that immediately after child birth the body becomes cold and it needs to remain hot and so this is given. Ras Sindoor is give to the child in half an hour's time immediately after birth, it is a root of one tree and is crushed and made into a dust and the child is given this so that he/she will never get fever and cold. After cord cutting mustard oil is applied and no medicine is given. Dai gives bath to the child immediately with hot water and 9 days later another bath is given after naming ceremony. Generally, the child is breast-fed till he is 3 years old.

TRADITIONAL CONTRACEPTIVE PRACTICES

(a) Disease Concept—As Narrated by Paadum and Doman Baskey

Diagnosis of any disease according to the Santhals is based on the examination of urine. Generally, the urine of the patient/ sick person is taken in a plate, further to this Mustard (*Sarso*) oil is added to it, this results into changing of urine into different colours and the urine moves into different directions with finally settling down in one location of the plate. Based on the location and colour of the urine in the plate, the traditional healer diagnoses if the person is suffereing from a disease called "*Pidiha*" in which the abdomen becomes tight only on the left side and there is too much of pain, the disease is mainly stones, and mostly occurs in small children who eat a lot of soil and mud, this has to be treated immediately otherwise the belief is that the stomach will burst.

Most of the medicines are developed and prepared out of plants, animal parts and minerals; e.g in case of *Pidiha* the medicine is prepared out of skin of an animal called *Bajar Kabti*, a smaller version of crocodile, a chameleon. The skin of chameleon is removed with stone and then it is powdered into a dust, this dust is mixed into water and the patient is given this paste as medicine.

Similarly, many such problems which the infants suffer from are understood differently, e.g. in case of colic pain, it is felt that blood is not circulating well in the body of the child and hence a mixture of *Jyeshta madha*, *Mishri chini* and *Mahua* leaves – *Boro* tree – is made finely and then is converted into tablets and given to the child to ensure good circulation of blood.

(b) Therapies for Stopping Conception and Pregnancies Completely

Sura, Nakhal, Hingu, Tutiya are powdered together and then converted to small tablets, which are then put into capsules, the women are given 3 times for 3 days consecutively, the intake of medicine results into bleeding which is black in color. Second month onwards the bleeding becomes normal.

Traditional Contraceptives

Traditional contraceptive methods have always been considered safe and effective by Santhals and have been commonly used. “The latest and probably the best modern reference about medicinal plants is James A. Duke’s Handbook of Medicinal Herbs (1985). Duke reports on twenty-seven contraceptive plants, but of there only eight are in Dioscorides.” Based on the anti-fertility response evoked by neem oil, polyherbal neem in a cream preparation showed contraceptive efficacy on intra-vaginal application and its safety was shown in monkeys (Garg et al 1993).

Neem oil acts as a spermicidal agent and inhibits sperm motility (Riar et al 1990; Sharma et al 1996). Several plant products have been tested for their anti-fertility activity at the University of Rajasthan. Lohiya et al (1990) showed that the hypokalemic effects of gossypol acetic acid could be reversed by concurrent use of potassium chloride. Chinoy et al (1984) showed the anti-fertility effects of crude extracts of Carica papaya seeds. Using crude aqueous and chloroform extracts of C. papaya seeds, sterile matings were recorded in rodents by Lohiya and Goyal (1992) and Lohiya et al (1999). The extracts immobilised human sperm *in vitro*, in a dose-dependent manner (Lohiya et al 2000a). A combination of the plant products i.e. Piper longum, Embelia ribes and Borax has been found to be effective as female contraceptive that has been tested through clinical trial.

(c) Initiative of *Sambandh* in Identification of Tradtional Contraceptive Practice

Sambandh has been involved in the process of promotion of indigenous health practice in Orissa since more than a decade. During this period we had came across more than 1500 traditional health practitioners of different parts of Orissa. The traditional health practitioners use different traditional methods as contraceptives. The different birth control methods used by the traditional healers are documented and these methods need more assessment and research to prove its efficacy.

(d) Contraceptives and Abortion inducing Herbs

1. *Abrus precatorius L:* Family with Collection Number – FABACEAE/225

   Vernacular Name - *Kaicho,Kaincho,Lalgunj,Runjo* (O,Ba,Bh,Su);*Gujjbai,Arakeej*,(Sa); *Karjani* (K); *Kouch, Ked, Ara-kuch* (Lo)

   Parts Used - White seeds

   Method of treatment: White seeds kept in unboiled cow milk for the period of over night and the seed is given to woman in the morning at the end of menstruation cycle for preventing conception.

2. *Annona squamosa L:* Family with Collection Number - (ANNONACEAE)/222

   Vernacular Name - Maghua,Ata, (O,Ba,Bh); *Boror - daru* (Lo); *Newa,Mondal* (Sa);
   Nenwa, Mandal (Ko)

Parts Used - Dried root powder

Ethno-medicinal use—For abortion of pregnancy: Dried root powder (5gm) is taken once in morning for five days by women for abortion of 3 to 4 months of pregnancy.

3. *Annona reticulata L:* Family with Collection Number - (ANNONACEAE) /320

   Vernacular Name - *Rajamaghua, Ramphala, Barhial,* (O,Ba,Bh); *Naga-newa, Ramphal*(Lo); *Mandargam, Gom* (Sa).

   Parts Used - Seed powder

   Ethno-medicinal use—For spoiling of pregnancy: A mixture of seed powder with black pepper (*Piper nigrum*) (about 3gm) is prescribed for spoiling of pregnancy up to 3-4 months duration.

4. *Borassus flabellifer L:* Family with Collection Number - (ARECACEAE)/260

   Vernacular Name - *Tala, Tal, Talo,* (O,Ba,Su,Bh); *Tar* (Sa); *Rola-daru* (Lo).

   Parts used - Male infloresence

   Ethno-medicinal use—as contraceptive: Ash (after burning of male infloresence) with powder of black peppers (*Piper longum*) and cow milk in the ratio of 2:1:1,is prescribed to women as contraceptive.

5. *Crateva nurvala Buch-Ham:* Family with Collection Number - (CAPPARACEAE)/344; Vernacular Name - *Barun, Varuna, Pitmaiel* (O,Ba); *Banena-ba* (Sa); *Barun daru* (Lo); Parts used - Stem bark

   Ethno-medicinal use—For contraceptive: Fresh juice of stem bark (3ml) mixed with seed powder of *Piper nigrum* (1gm) is taken by women in the seventh days of menstrual cycle as a contraceptive.

6. *Hibiscus rosa-sinensis L:* Family with Collection Number - (MALVACEAE)./346.

Vernacular Name - *Parijat, Mondaro, Mandar* (O,Ba); *Jaba-gacha* (Lo,Mu,Sa).

Parts Used - Stem bark

Ethno-medicinal use—as Contraceptive: Stem bark paste (15gm) is given to woman continuously five days for causing abortion and mixture of pasty mass of flower buds (3gm) with rust of iron (2gm) and country liquor (2ml) is taken by women at the days of menstruation as a contraceptive.

For gaining vitality; avoiding post-natal complications; easing the delivery process

1. *Dillenia aurea Sm:* Family with Collection Number—DILLE NIACEAE) /136.

   Vernacular Name - *Rai,* (O,Ba); *Rai-daru*,(Lo); *Korkotta* (Sa,Ko).

   Parts Used-Stem bark

   Ethno-medicinal use—Gaining of vitality after child birth: Extract of stem bark (10ml) is taken once a day for two week in empty stomach for restoration of health after child birth.

2. *Dillenia pentagyna Roxb:* Family with Collection Number - (DILLE NIACEAE) /231, Vernacular Name - *Rai*(O,Ko,Bh); *Aghai* (Mu); *Sahar*, *Korkota* (Mu).

   Parts Used - Stem bark

   Ethno-medicinal use—For easy delivery: Midwives (*Dhai*) of ethnic group uses tree gum for easy delivery purpose.

3. *Tephrosia purpurea (L.) Pers.:* Family Collection Number - (FABACEAE). /304

   Vernacular Name - *Bano-kuthi, Gileri, Kulathio, Ban-nilo, Mohisia-Kotathiya, Pokha, Soropokha, Kulathia* (O,Ba,Su); *Nol-gach, Bir-chakunda* (Lo); *Anuraida* (Sa).

   Parts Used - Leaf

   Ethno-medicinal use—For post natal complications: Decoction of leaf (5ml) mixed with honey (2ml) given to women twice a day continuously for one month against post-natal complications.

4. *Tephrosia purpurea (L.) Pers.:* Family with Collection Number FABACEAE). /304. Vernacular Name: *Bano-kuthi, Gileri, Kulathio, Ban-nilo, Mohisia-Kotathiya, Pokha, Soropokha, Kulathia* (O, Ba, Su); *Nol-gach, Bir-chakunda* (Lo); *Anuraida* (Sa).

   Parts Used: Leaf

   Ethno-medicinal use: Decoction of leaf (5ml) mixed with honey (2ml) given to women twice a day continuously for one month against post-natal complications.

(e) Herbs for Secretion of Breast Milk

1. *Ficus hispida L.f. Suupl.:* Family with Collection Number - (MORACEAE)./366.

   Vernacular Name - *Panidimiri, Demburu, Kharsen, Dimiri, Baidimiri,* (O,Ba); *Duma* (Sa); *Kosta* (Lo).

   Parts Used - Fruit

   Ethno-medicinal use—For Milk secretion: Boiled green fruits given to mother as a glactogogue for better milk. Hadarachua (Sa); Kantagadi (Ba); Badajhada (Mu).

(f) Herbs for Treating Impotency and Arousing Sexual Desire

1. *Phyla nodiflora (L.) Greene:* Family with Collection Number - (VERBENACEAE). /318. Vernacular Name - *Gosingi,* (O,Ba,Su); *Jalapipla* (Sa).

   Parts Used - Root

   Ethno-medicinal use—For promoting sexual desire: Decoction of root (3ml) with unboiled egg (2mg) is given to women to promote sexual desire.

2. *Momordica charantia L:* Family with Collection Number—(CUCURBITACEAE)./131. Vernacular Name: *Kalara, Kolera,* (O, Ba, Su, Bh); Koradi (Sa & Mu).

   Parts Used: Fruit

Ethno-medicinal use: Fruit juice (3ml) mixed with root paste of *Hemidesmus indicus* (2gm) is taken twice a day after food for one month against sex debility.

3. *Phyla nodiflora (L.) Greene:* Family with Collection Number - (VERBENACEAE). /318; Vernacular Name: *Gosingi,* (O, Ba, Su); Jalapipla (Sa).

   Parts Used: Root

   Ethno-medicinal use: Decoction of root (3ml) with un boiled egg (2mg) is given to women to promote sexual desire. *Gadiapala* (Sa); *Ashanabani* (Ba, Su); *Kaliasahi* (Ko).

4. *Withania somnifera L:* Family with Collection Number—(SOLANACEAE)./242; Vernacular Name: *Ashwagandha* (O, Ba, Su); *Care-su* (Lo).

   Parts Used: Flower

   Ethno-medicinal use: Decoction of flower with honey is taken in the ratio of frequently for one month against seminal weakness.

(g) Herbs for Treating Irregular Menstruation and Anaemia

1. *Bombax ceiba L.:* Family with Collection Number - (BOMBACACEAE)/.231

   Vernacular Name: *Semulo, Simili, Simal* (O, Ba, Bh); *Simal-dare, Daldara* (Sa, Ko); *Edel-daru* (Lo)

   Parts used: Fleshy roots

   Ethno-medicinal use: Paste of fleshy roots of young plant (1 gm) mixed with unboiled cow milk (2ml) is taken once a day in the early morning for a week by women to regulate irregular menstruation and flowers paste is apply on boils before bed for ripening purpose. *Noto* (Lo); *Kotoria* (Ba); *Kaptipada* (Sa).

2. *Heliotropium indicum L.:* Family with Collection Number - (BORAGINACEAE)./250

   Vernacular Name: *Hati-sura* (Lo); *Hatisundha* (O, Ba, Su, Go).

Parts Used: Root

Ethno-medicinal use: Root paste (3mg) with lime is used by rubbing the infected portion of skin as a cure for ring worms and decoction of root (10ml) with honey (2ml) is taken as vitamin for iron deficiency by woman against anaemia during pregnancy period.

3. *Triticum aestivum L.:* Family with Collection Number - (POACEAE)./245

   Vernacular Name: *Gahama, Gonhu*, (O, Ba, Su); *Goin, Gahu* (Lo & Sa).

   Parts Used: oil of the ghost

   Ethno-medicinal use: Wheat bran oil (5ml) with country liquor (3ml) is prescribed to girls for treatment of dysmenorrhoea (painful menstruation).

While the adolescent girls have incessant periods from day 1 to 10 or many times irregular periods, or at times if its completely black then it is understood that there is some disorder and in such cases a mixture of *Jyeshtha Madha* along with *Mahua Leaves*, *Basang* leaves and golden *bhasma* is prepared and is converted into tablets. If menses do not come then it is understood as though there are stones in the reproductive tract and hence there is mostly pain in the evenings, because the body has become cold. In such a case the parts of *Chayli* tree are given with lime, it is then understood that the blood gets boiled and the pain reduces.

The use of traditional medicine for gynaecological disorders is widespread in this region with higher percentage of the population relying on it. The study revealed that whatever knowledge on plants exists with the people of Mayurbhanj district, they are on fast declining because lack of interest of local youth to learn the traditional knowledge from the old herbal healer. The highly interesting findings for gynaecological disorder require further research, while the efficacy of the various indigenous practices will need to be subjected to pharmacological validation. Therefore, greater efforts are required to document traditional knowledge of the local people so as to prepare a comprehensive account of it, which will open new vistas in plant research which is much more safe, less costly and eco-friendly.

Herbal medicine has been widely practised throughout the world since ancient times. These medicines are safe and environmentally friendly. According to WHO about 80 per cent of the world's population relies on traditional medicine for their primary health care. India, being one of the world's 12 mega biodiversity countries, enjoys export of herbal raw material worth U.S. $100-114 million per year approximately. Currently the Government of India, realising the value of the country's vast range of medicinal plants, has embarked on a mission of documenting the traditional knowledge about medicinal plants and herbs.

The local uses of plants as a cure are common particularly in those areas, which have little or no access to modern health services, such as the innumerable tribal villages and hamlets in India. The indigenous traditional knowledge of medicinal plants of various ethnic communities, where it has been transmitted orally for centuries is fast disappearing from the face of the earth due to the advent of modern technology and transformation of traditional culture.

6

Ethno-medical Practices Among Gonds

PROFILE OF GONDS

Origin/History

The Gonds are one of the most famous and important tribes in India, known for their unique customs and traditions. They are mainly a nomadic tribe and call themselves as *Koyathoria*. The term *'Gond'* is derived from the Telugu word *'Konda'* this means hill.

The Gonds are traditionally agriculturalists and some practice shifting cultivation even today. Other major activities of Gonds include collecting forest produce, fishing, hunting, forging metal goods in cottage industries and other primary sector activities. Gonds also have a special skill that has been passed down every generation and that is the secrets of the medicine plants. As there are no proper health facilities in several areas, they still follow the traditional system of medicines and use plants and herbs for curing various ailments. Gonds are also known for practising social hierarchy system like Hindus and the Gond society is regarded as highly stratified and not conforming to the usual image of egalitarianism among tribals.

The Gonds have gained enormous popularity for their unique and distinct social customs and traditions and have become the subject of great interest among sociologists and researchers all over the world. The main language of the Gonds is *Gondi* but about half of Gond populations also speak Indo-Aryan dialects including Hindi. The Gondi language is related to Telugu and other Dravidian languages.

There exists little known history of the Gonds, and it was not until the Mughal times that Gonds figured in contemporary chronicles. But the ruins of forts ascribed to Gond Rajas suggest that Gonds in the past did not believe in solitary existence as believed to be practiced by other tribes. Until comparatively recent times, a feudal system prevailed also in the lands of Adilabad, and myths and epics depict the life of Gond chieftains who were not subject to any outside power. The Gonds were already settled agriculturalists who cultivated their land with plough and bullocks by around 1970s. Land was plentiful, and individuals could move freely from one settlement to another. This mobility has now come to an end, and with this the entire life-style of the Gonds has changed.

Although regarded as tribals, the Gonds, or *Koyathor*, as they call themselves, have a rich legendary history. In the fourteenth century they were the ruling class in many parts of central India. During this time several small Gond kingdoms were consolidated by Gond kings to form a Gond dynasty. They built numerous palaces, forts, tanks and lakes, but were overcome by Muslim armies in 1592. Towards the end of the eighteenth century the Gonds had scattered into many tribes.

They believe in the existence of gods and spirits, both benevolent and malevolent. The song here is sung at the death of a person beseeching the spirit of the dead to stop troubling the living. It is based on the Kondh belief that people love their homes so much that their souls are reluctant to leave the hearth even after death.

These spirits, though generally kind, can become harmful at times since they are now unable to participate in earthly life. It is, therefore, customary to make generous offerings to the spirit. The song begins by saying that the dead spirit will be able to receive offerings only if the others in the family continue to live and prosper. They reveal their willingness to do anything to make the spirit happy but, in return, the spirit must also promise not to trouble them with its visits.

The Gonds, like the other Tribals of central India, believe that most diseases and misfortunes are caused by the machinations of evil spirits and offended deities. It is the task of the soothsayers and diviners to find out which supernatural agencies have caused the present sickness or misfortune and how they can be appeased. If soothsayers and diviners cannot help, magicians and shamans must be employed. Magicians believe that by magic formulas and devices they can force a particular deity or spirit to carry out their commands. Shamans are persons who easily fall into trances and are then believed to be possessed by deities or spirits that prophesy through their mouths. These frequent ecstasies do not seem to have any detrimental mental or physical effects on the shamans, who may be male or female. Magic may be "white" or "black": it is white if it counteracts black magic or effects a cure when a sickness has been caused by black magic. Gonds also believe in the evil eye and in witchcraft. A witch is usually a woman who by her evil power brings sickness and death to people in the neighbourhood. When discovered, she is publicly disgraced and expelled from the village or even killed.

"Gond poetry is simple and symbolic, free of all literary conventions and allusions. It is poetry of earth and sky, of forest, hill and river, of the changing seasons and the varied passions of men, poetry of love, naked and unashamed, unchecked by any inhibition or restraint. The bulk of the poems are songs of the dance and the most poetic of them are perhaps the songs of the great *Karma* dance which is common to many of the primitive tribes of Central India. This dance symbolises the growth of the green branches of the forest in the spring: sometimes a tree is set up in the village and the people dance around it. The men leap forward to a rapid roll of drums and the women sway back before them. Then bending low to the ground, the women dance, their feet moving in perfect rhythm until the group of singers advances towards them like the steady urge of wind coming and going among the tree tops and the girls swing to and fro in answer. They often dance all night until lost in a lapture of movement, they surprise the secret of Lila, the ecstasy of creation, that ancient zest in the glory of which God made all things".

Geographical Distribution

Gond tribes are primarily located in Madhya Pradesh, Chhattisgarh, eastern Maharashtra, northern Andhra Pradesh and western Orissa. With a population of over 4 millions, Gonds also form the largest tribal group in central India. In Chhattisgarh, Gonds are the largest tribal group in terms of population and are mainly concentrated in the southern part of the state. More than 20 per cent of Gonds in Chhattisgarh live in Bastar region only. There are 3 major sub-castes of Gonds in Bastar—Maria, Muria and Dorla.

To the people of northern India it was known as Gondwāna, an unexplored country of inaccessible mountains and impenetrable forests, inhabited by the savage tribes of Gonds from whom it took its name. Hindu kingdoms were, it is true, established over a large part of its territory in the first centuries of our era, but these were not accompanied by the settlement and opening out of the country, and were subsequently subverted by the Dravidian Gonds, who perhaps invaded the country in large numbers from the south between the ninth and twelfth centuries. Hindu immigration and colonisation from the surrounding provinces occurred at a later period, largely under the encouragement and auspices of Gond kings. Many Gonds live around the Satpura Hills, Maikala Range and Son-Deogarh uplands, and on the Bastar plateau. Many Gond tribes also live in the Garhjat Hills of northern Orissa.

Sub-tribes

Gonds have nearly 45-50 clans (sub-tribe) spread over several districts. The clans are usually named after some animals or plants. Among the common clans in Chhattisgarh are Markam (mango tree), Tekam (teak tree), and Netam (the dog) and so on. From these animals and plants a clan derives its name and totems for the members of its social group. The totemic association generally has a legendary background. Gonds are also different types of division. And division is of thirteen types: (i) Raj Gond; (ii) Koytilya Gond; (iii) Raghuwal Gond; (iv) Padal Gond; (v) Ozyal Gond; (vi) Dholi Gond; (vii) Thotyal Gond; (viii) Maria Gond; (ix) Koikopal Gond; (x) Muria Gond; (xi) Mari Gond; (xii) Rawanvasi Gond; (xiii) Kolan Gond.

Religious Beliefs

If a Gond, when starting on a journey in the morning, meets a tiger, cat or hare or a four horned deer, he returns and postpones his journey, but if he meets one of these animals when he is well on the way it is considered to be lucky. Rainfall at a wedding on some other festival is unlucky, as it is believed to be someone's cry.

When there is drought two boys put a pestle across their shoulders, tie a living frog to it with a rag, and go from house to house accompanied by other boys and girls singing "*Mendak Bhai Pani De*" (Brother Frog give rain). The frog is considered to be able to produce rain because it lives in water and therefore has control over its elements. Burial of the dead has probably been the general custom of the Gonds in the past, and the introduction of cremation may be ascribed to Hindu influence.

The festivals of Gonds are not so much associated with religion as is the case with most Hindu festivals. Their festivals are in response to the harvest season and local customs. Due to their frequent contact with Hindu population, their folk-ways are now becoming apparently tinged with the colour of Hinduism.Gonds observes many Hindu festivals without understanding their religious significance. Most celebrations consist of offerings to Gods, feast drinking and dancing. On the whole, their festivals tend to be recreational rather than spiritual.

Their festivals are also connected with agricultural cycle. Their enthusiasm and zeal depends upon the success of harvest. Festivals are the only occasions in which Gonds ever indulge in any extravagance, otherwise they believe only in securing two square meals. Throughout the year a number of fairs, festivals and feasts are organised in the village. However, their distribution over a year is rather irregular: (i) *Hareli:* Hareli is the festival of rain. It is observed in the early period of rains. The goddess of crop '*Kutki Dai*' is worshipped on this occasion to ensure better harvest. This is mostly in the month of July-August. '*Hareli*' word is probably derived from Hindi word, 'Haryali' which means greenery as in this seasons vegetations begins to bloom and there is greenery all around; (ii) *Khyania:* In the month of August seven days before 'Rakhi; Gonds sow the wheat grains in the *Tukania* . On the next day of Rakhi i.e after 8 days they cut the wheat crop from the basket. They exchange this with one another. Some of it is also immersed in the water on the same day. Gonds estimate the success or failure of crop of coming season by this festival; (iii) *Rakhi:* On the day of Rakhi Gond women imitating the Hindu customs tie string around the wrist of their brothers and cousins for their safety, security and protection; (iv) *Dashera:* It is observed in the month of October and is quite an important festival among Gonds. But unlike a Hindu festival, it is not associated with any Hindus rites or religious beliefs. Its importance is mainly due to the agricultural ceremony attached to it. During this month the spells of rain ends and active agricultural seasons sets in the villages.

Gonds indulge in heavy drinking, throw feasts. Saila and Reena dances are the common features of the festivals; (v) *Mela Madai:* It is held after the completion of the harvesting of the paddy crop, when the people are free from their agricultural work and their stores are full with grain. After Diwali this fair is enjoyed daily for a week. The head of the village inaugurates the Mela. People light oil lamps at their houses. They dance and sing day and night. This celebration is made in the happiness of the success of their harvest. Sweet dishes and special food items are prepared in Gond houses on this occasion; (vi) *Nawa Feast:* In this festival, harvest thanking is celebrated. New harvested rice is offered to 'Budha Dev' under a Saj Tree for the first time new rice is cooked in the house, by the head of the family who has to keep fast on that day. On this occasion womenfolk do not cook rice; (vii) *Holi:* It is a spring festival. In the month of March, Holi is celebrated. It is a five day festival. A Gond will never miss the opportunity of drinking alcohol during Holi. On the first day of Holi festivals they play with '*kecher*' . Holi mela is also held during these days. It is merely a social recreation for Gonds which they have adopted from the local Hindu people.

The Gonds worship an animal god called *Ghaturiya* (sankat mochan), a reptile that climbs the trees and mountains very fast and hence they call it a god that has strength of climbing.

The religion of the Gonds does not differ much from that of the numerous other tribes in central India. Like them, the Gonds believe in a high god whom they call either by his Hindu name, "*Bhagwan*," or by his tribal name, "*Bara Deo*," the "Great God." But he is an otiose deity and is rarely worshiped, though his name is often invoked. He is a personal god—eternal, just, merciful, maker of the fertile earth and of man—though the universe is conceived as coexisting with him. In the Gond belief system, besides this high god there also exist a great number of male and female deities and spirits that personify various natural features. Every hill, river, lake, tree, and rock is inhabited by a spirit. The earth, water, and air are ruled by deities that must be venerated and appeased with sacrifices and offerings. These deities and spirits may be benevolent, but often they are capricious, malevolent, and prone to harming human beings, especially individuals who have made themselves vulnerable by breaking a rule of the tribal code. The deities and spirits, especially the ancestor spirits, watch over the strict observance of the tribal rules and punish offenders.

Gonds distinguish between priests and magicians. The village priest is appointed by the village council; however, his appointment is often hereditary. His responsibility is to perform all the sacrifices held at certain feasts for the village community for which he receives a special remuneration. Sacrifices and religious ceremonies on family occasions are usually performed by the head of the family. The diviners and magicians, on the other hand, are unofficial charismatic intermediaries between the supernatural world and human beings. The Gonds, like the other Tribals of central India, believe that most diseases and misfortunes are caused by the machinations of evil spirits and offended deities. It is the task of the soothsayers and diviners to find out which supernatural agencies have caused the present sickness or misfortune and how they can be appeased. If soothsayers and diviners cannot help, magicians and shamans must be employed. Magicians believe that by magic formulas and devices they can force a particular deity or spirit to carry out their commands.

Shamans are persons who easily fall into trances and are then believed to be possessed by deities or spirits that prophesy through their mouths. These frequent ecstasies do not seem to have any detrimental mental or physical effects on the shamans, who may be male or female. Magic may be "white" or "black": it is white if it counteracts black magic or effects a cure when a sickness has been caused by black magic. Gonds also believe in the evil eye and in witchcraft. A witch is usually a woman who by her evil power brings sickness and death to people in the neighbourhood. When discovered, she is publicly disgraced and expelled from the village or even killed.

The gonds worship the sun and call him by different names in different regions, like Bara deo, Buddha deo – the great god also called as mahadeo and narayan deo who stays over saj tree in thickest portion of the forest and never leaves it, ghaagra deo the bell god, Pharsa pen – the battle axe god, sankara deo – the chain god, dulha deo – the bridegroom god, kodiyal – the horse god, matiya – the whirlwind god, hulera – the cattle god. Offerings are made of blood and can only be performed by the priests called pardhans or ojhas.

In other instances, the consumption of the body was similar to an act of purification in India, the Gonds were known to kidnap boys of the Brahmin caste, kill them and sprinkle their blood over the fields in an attempt to placate the gods. Although such practices may seem barbaric, they are no different and no less illogical than many religious practices even today.

Hereditary bards and professional storytellers called Pardhans tell stories about Gond legends and myths. This makes for a rich oral tradition. In these stories, it is said that when Gond gods were born, their mother abandoned them. The goddess Parvati rescued them, but her consort Sri Shambhu Mahadeo (Shiva) kept them captive in a cave. Pahandi Kapar Lingal, a Gond hero, who received help from the goddess Jangu Bai, rescued them from the cave. They came out of the cave in four groups, thus laying the foundations of the basic four fold division of Gond society. Lingal also is responsible for creating a Gond kinship system and establishing a group of great Gond gods.

Persa Pen is the most distinctive feature of Gond religion. Like many other tribes, Gonds worship a high god known as Baradeo, whose alternate names are Bhagavan, Sri Shambu Mahadeo, and Persa Pen. Baradeo oversees activities of lesser gods. He is respected but he does not receive fervent devotion, which is shown only to clan deities. Each Gond clan has its Persa Pen, who protects all clan members. The Persa Pen is essentially good but can be dangerous and violent. Many Gonds believe that when a Pardhan (bard) plays his fiddle, the deity and fierce powers can be controlled.

Gond Dances

All Gonds are very fond of dancing. It is the great amusement of the people. Night after night in the eastern tracts in the cool, moon-lit nights of the hot weather, the sojourner in the camp is lulled to sleep by the rhythmic lilt of a Gondi chorus as the villagers dance round a fire in some open space near the hamlet. The favourite dance is a peculiar rippling step forward with the foot dragged, not very graceful when done by a single individual, but looking quite different when done in unison by a great circle of dancers singing a 're-la', 're-la', chorus to which the step keeps time. In some villages, where the headman is an enthusiast for the pastime, a trained band performs weird and wonderful step dances to the sound of the drum. At a big dance, the trained band occupies the inner ring round the fire, while the common folk, men and maids, in separate rings move round in great circles in opposite ways. All are dressed for the occasion in their best, bearing in their hands weird ornaments of wicker work, with garlands of flowers on their necks and in their hair, feather ornaments humorously or coquettishly placed. Seen in the glow of a huge log fire, glinting on the shining beads and barbaric ornaments of the dancers, with the throb of the drums and the beat of many feet moving in unison to the wild music of the voices in chorus, a Madia dance is a spectacle not easily forgotten, but lingers as a characteristic scene when other details have faded out of the memory. Men and women ordinarily dance in separate circles but in the dances where the young men choose their brides, they dance in couples.

Clans

Gond society is divided into four groups known as *phratries* or *sagas* in Gondi. Each saga traces its descent to one of the four groups of gods who emerged from the cave after their release by the hero Lingal. The saga is divided into several clans *(pari)*. A clan consists of a group of people who believe they share a common ancestor. Generally, it is good to marry outside the clan.

Family Type

Kinship terms used by different castes and groups are almost the same all over the state except with little difference in their pronunciation. Kutumb (means family) is the smallest unit that shares the common rituals and the mores of the clan. All the members of the family unit are bound by a kinship tie. Patriarchal system prevails in the state. Hence, the elder son inherits the father's right and property. The tribals are no exception to this practice. The position of a wife in a Kutumb depends upon her husband; that of the mother is recognised in relation to her children. Sex, age and supporting capacity of an individual are the deciding factors which govern his role in the family. Without a male child a family is considered incomplete. Widows and divorced daughters of a family are accepted as liabilities. Separation from a Kutumb in the same village or town is not encouraged. It is contrarily taken improper if somebody ventures to break the ties with a joint family. Then there are ways in which people are linked through ritual acts. One of such kinships is the kinship of ritual brothers and sisters, known as gurubhai and gurubahen, which is acquired through a common teacher. This type of kinship is regarded more serious in the dharma sambandha—the relation sanctioned by religion. The duties attached to this form of kinship are mostly the same as performed in real kin tie.

Majority of these have been traditionally been described as Raj Gonds, though in their own language they call themselves Koitur, a word common to most Gondi Dialects. The term Raj Gonds, widely used even in 1940s has now become obsolete, thanks to the political eclipse of the Gond Rajas.

Gond society has both vertical stratification and horizontal divisions, and while the decline of the Rajas has led to the decline of stratification based on hereditary rank, the division of society based on exogamous patrilineal units has retained its importance. The basis of social structure is a system of four phratries, each divided into sub-clans, and the origin of this structure is attributed to a divine cultural hero. The members of each clan worship a diety called *persa pen* (great god) and in some case the shrine of this deity lies within the ancestral clan land.

The Gonds have a traditional tribal council known as the panchayat and each group has its own traditional panchayat. These councils are headed by a mukhiya, and a few others assist him. As long as they perform their duties effectively, fresh elections do not take place. The primary purpose of these panchayats is to maintain peace and harmony in respective villages and safeguard and uphold Gond customs.

Gonds welcome visitors with dried tobacco leaves, fruits, or other small gifts. Many villages have guest huts.

Marriage

Gonds follow tribal endogamy and clan exogamy. Monogamous marriage is common among the Gonds. Cross cousin marriage is preferred. They fallow the system of patriarchy. Both men and women used to be tattooed earlier but this is constantly on decline among men. The clans are usually named after some animals or plants. The religious observances include prohibitions against members of the totemic group, killing or eating the totemic species. The worship of ancestors is an integral part of their religion. Budha Deo, the great God, was probably at first the Saj tree, but afterwards, the whole collections of gods were sometimes called Budha Deo. They believe also in numbers of local deities. The Gonds have a highly developed aesthetic sense.

The position of women among Gonds is practically that of equality with the other sex. Normally a Gond maid is free to be wooed by the man of her choice and hardly any girl is under sixteen at the time of marriage. The young couple generally first agree to be married but the negotiations are carried on by their elders. When a betrothal has been arranged, the bridegroom's party comes and plants a spear in the courtyard of the bride's house which none may pull up. If the bride's party consent, water is poured over the spear by the father of the girl and the ceremony may then proceed. Should the bride's father fail to do this, the bridegroom's party considers itself insulted and the father of the bride is heavily fined. A platform of cowdung cakes is built on which a blanket is spread; on this the couple takes its stand and exchange vows. The bridegroom puts an iron ring on the finger of the bride and the ceremony is complete. The pair then leaves the wedding party and betakes itself to a temporary but previously prepared rendezvous in the forest.

When a man is unable to pay the bride-price demanded by the parent, it is sometimes arranged that he serves the parent for his bride. A parent may demand five, eight or ten year's service. If during the first three years the bride is not known to have lost her chastity, the full marriage ceremony then takes place, but it the contrary is proved the marriage takes place by *pat* ceremony. In *pat* or widow marriage the pair stands under the eaves of the bridegroom's house with an upright spear between them. A mixture of turmeric and oil is applied to the bridegroom's fore-head and to the iron spearhead. A string of beads is then tied round the neck of the bride by the bridegroom and the pair walks into the house man and wife.

In marriage by capture, the bridegroom collects a party of friends and carries off the bride from her village. When they arrive at the bridegroom's house, a pot of water is poured over their heads and they become man and wife but are supposed to live apart until the full marriage ceremony can be performed.

Marriage by capture has fallen into disuse as it was apt to lead to complications with the Indian Penal Code. But irrespective of the Code, it was not free from difficulty. Major Lucie Smith records a case wherein a fascinating Gond maid of 16 was carried off from her village and married to suitor No. I. Next night a disappointed rival's party appeared and carried her off and married her to suitor No. II. Then her own village party arose to ask as to whose wife she was and the young woman solved the difficulty by declaring for suitor No. I. There remained the delicate question as to whether she was to be married with *marmi,* the full wedding ceremony or *pat,* second marriage, rites. It was finally decided by the elders that only *pat* rites could be granted, which was certainly very hard on the young woman.

Talking about gender and other elations, both types of cross cousin marriages are prevalent among the Gonds, i.e. marriage with the father's sister's daughter, or marriage with the mother's brother's daughter. The most common type of marriage is by negotiation and is commonly called Biwa, while there are other modes of acquiring a mate like marriage by exchange (Sattabata Biwa), marriage by service (Oharjawai Biwa) and marriage by intrusion (Charningni Biwa). Bride Price in cash and kind is generally paid to the Bride's father, and monogyny is the general practice, though polygamy is permitted.

Marriages are preferred within blood relation. Their men have to pay a bridal price to the father of the bride. In case a man is unable to afford a particular woman, he can negotiate the price. Some prefer to work in the brides home for sometime till the time it is equivalent to the bride price. In case of death of the husband she can marry his younger or elder brother but has to be unmarried. Gond tribals of Baster have their own system Ghotul in which unmarried boys and girls can live together in separately made huts where others are not allowed. During this time can change their partners for their best gratification. They dance, sing, drink and exchange knowledge. If they want they can leave and go for marriage.

Gonds believe that a person's soul neither goes to heaven nor rests in peace if he has not married a virgin. But those who do not find virgins at times marry widows or divorced woman. When a Gond man marries second time, no elaborate ceremonies are observed. An elderly woman of the house performs a ceremony of haldi-dalna and churi-pahanana. A second wife can be brought in the presence of first wife, or after the death of first wife or after divorce. This ceremony is called as Char-bathana. Gonds fallow tribal endogamy and clan exogamy. Gond consider monogamy as the ideal type and prefer to have only one wife at a given moment of time except in certain exceptional circumstances, for example, cases where the wife is barren. A Gond is expected to marry his cross-cousin except in certain circumstances. Strict adherence to this custom results in many unhappy unions, elopements and divorce in the community.

Cross cousin marriage is locally termed as *doodh-lautana*, while literally meaning, 'to return the milk'— an act of reciprocity on the part of an individual among the Gonds. The custom has strong socio-religious force behind it. Thus, a Gond male may marry either his mother's brother's daughter (Mo Bo Da) or father's sister's daughter (Fa Si Da).

Marriage with mother's-brother's-daughter is called s *doodh-duhani* vivah and with father's sister's daughter as *Pal-duhani vivah*. While cross cousin marriage is preferred, the incidence of any parallel cousin marriage has not been observed. Patriarchy prevails in this community. The Gond believe in a number of Gods (Dev) like Teen devki, Chardevki, Panchdevki and Satdevki—which are considered as sub-totemic on sub-clan groups. Clans worshipping with sub totem, for example Chardevki constitute one samdhan (a corporate group) and has to seek spouses for their sons and daughters from the clan of another samdhan group. The members of one samdhan group refer each other as brother and sisters. Hence, a marriage between them is a social taboo. If such a union takes place, it is considered a breach of incest taboo by community and the couple is ostracised (hated) by the community.

Diet

The staples of the Gond diet are two millets known as *kodo* and *kutki*. These are either boiled to a broth or cooked to a dry cereal. Broth is preferred for the first two meals of the day and the dry cereal is eaten at night, often with vegetables. Vegetables are either grown in gardens or collected from forests along with roots and tubers. Honey is also gathered from forests. Rice is a luxury item that Gonds enjoy during feasts and festivals. Most Gonds like meat. Animals sacrificed at ceremonies are eagerly consumed, and animals hunted in the forest supplement the diet. Gonds must abstain from the flesh of animals that are their clan totems.

Gonds grow tobacco for smoking and for celebrations make liquor from the mahua tree.

Birth Rituals/Ceremonies

Gonds protect pregnant women against spells and evil influences, and perform several rituals after a baby is born. A mother's brother generally names a baby boy, while the father's sister names a girl. Children grow up as part of a family, clan, and *phratry* (one of the four main divisions of Gond society), and gradually learn the ways of their people. Both boys and girls help guard family crops from birds and monkeys. Males undergo a ritual shaving of the beard, mustache, and eyebrows as a sign of adulthood. Girls are considered full-grown at their first menstruation.

On the 9th day after the birth of a child, a feast is given and the naming ceremony takes place. It may he named after the month or the season as *Wanja* from *Wanji,* rice *i.e.,* one born in the rice harvest or *Irpa* trom *irpu,* the *mahua* flower. Should a difficulty occur about a name, a little rice is tied in a piece of cloth and swung in trout of the child while a list of names is shouted out. At whatever name the child clutches the cloth that name is chosen. After the birth of the first son, the names of the parents are merged in the name of the son. Thus if the son be called Reka, the father is known as Rekaltapa and the mother as Rekaltanni.

In a Gond community if a child is born with his feet first, its feet are supposed to have special power, and people suffering from pain in the back come and have their backs touched by the toes of the child's left foot. This power is believed to be retained in later life of the child too. The diseases of children are attributed to evil sprits. The illness called sukhi in which the body and limbs grow weak and have a dried up appearance, is very common and is probably caused by malnutrition. They attribute it to the machination of an owl which has heard the child's name or obtained a piece of its soiled clothing. In order to cure this illness they use charms and amulets, and also let the child wallow in a pig-sty so that it may become as fat as pig.

If a child is taking a long time before learning to speak, they give it leaves of the pipal tree to eat, because the leaves of this tree make a noise by rust-ling in the wind; or a root which is very light in weight, because they think that the tongue is heavy and the quality of lightness will thus be communicated to it. A child is given grain to eat for the first time six months after birth. The first teeth of a child are thrown on to the roof of the house, because the rats, who have especially good and sharp teeth, live there, and it is hoped that the child's second teeth may grow like theirs. Or they are placed under a water-pot in the hope that the child's second teeth may grow as fast as the grass does under water-pots. If a child is lean some people take it to a place where asses have lain down and rolled in ashes; they roll the child in the ashes similarly and believe that it will get fat like the asses are. Or they may lay the child in a pig-sty with the same idea. People who want to injure a child get hold of its coat and lay it out in the sun to dry, in the belief that the child's body will dry up in a similar manner.

Puberty Rituals/Ceremonies

Among the Gonds tribal groups, cross-cousin marriage is called "bringing back the milk," alluding to the gift of a girl in one generation being returned by the gift of a girl in the next.

Death Rituals

The Gonds tribes sometimes cremate and sometimes bury their dead bodies. Generally they bury those who die of small pox or leprosy. The dead person, whether male or female, is buried. He is buried with face upwards, head to the north and feet to the south, in clothes in which he died with, a new cloth spread over the body. The body is not given a bath before burial.

The dead are usually buried with the feet pointing to the North in opposition to the Hindu practice, and this fact has been adduced in evidence of the Gond's beliefs that their ancestors came from the North. The funeral takes place on the same day when the people assembled. Some pieces of cloth, together with him, so that they may accompany his sprit to the other world. Children who die when still at breast feeding stage are buried at the roots of a mahua tree, as it is thought that they will suck liquor from them and be nourished as if by their mother's milk.

Ceremonies are performed at the funeral to prevent the soul of the deceased from finding its way back to its house and village. The Gonds believe in an afterlife. They believe each human being has two souls, the life spirit and the shadow. The shadow must be prevented from returning to its home, or it will harm the surviving relatives. The life spirit goes to Bhagwan to be judged and rewarded by reincarnation into a higher form or punished in a pool of biting worms; after a while the soul is reborn and begins a new life. Others believe that the soul joins the other ancestors of the clan, especially after a stone memorial has been erected. Still others believe that the soul is absorbed in Bhagwan or Bara Deo. The belief in the survival of the ancestral spirits is, however, quite strong. These ancestor spirits watch over the moral behaviour of the living Gond and punish offenders of tribal law. Thus they act as strict guardians of the Gond community.

Children, unmarried persons, and individuals dying an inauspicious death (for instance, in an epidemic) are buried without much ceremony. Gonds believe humans have a life force and a spirit. On death, the life force is reincarnated into another earthly existence, but the spirit remains in the other world. Gonds perform death rituals to help the spirit move into the other world and to ease its acceptance by other clan spirits. This rite, known as *karun*, must be done to fulfill an obligation to the deceased. Memorial pillars honour the dead. Gonds believe ancestral spirits watch over the living, punish offenders, and guard Gond communities.

Persons who die of cholera or small-pox and young children are buried but others are usually burnt. The body is borne by the mourners to the burning place and laid on the pile of fire wood which is lighted. The skull of the deceased is broken with a stake which is specially placed for the purpose. The mourners then leave the pile and wash in a stream. An ox is sometimes killed, but more often a goat or fowl and the flesh eaten by the mourners. The animal must be slain by a single blow from a heavy wooden axe. After the feast the mourners return home and refrain for three days from their usual occupations. A small cromlech is built on the spot where the body was burnt and usually a pot with a few small coins is placed within it.

Soul Migration Rituals

One Gond belief is that the soul of the slain will inhibit the image of the tiger thus set up, and being inimical to his slayer will attack tiger at every opportunity and thus act as a village guardian. Once a year, a great pilgrimage of Gonds and other Hindus is made to Sat Bahini, the great flat-topped hill near Nagbhir; concerning which there are confused legends. The Gond believes in the immortality of the soul, but his faith is a very vague one. Amongst some transmigration is dimly held and a curious ceremony is performed which tends to define this belief. A Gond like most Indians must not die on a bed but stretched on Mother Earth. On the place where a man's head rested at the moment of death, a small head of grain is made and covered with a basket on which a lighted lamp is extinguished, the basket lifted and the wise among the Gond discern on the heap of grain, the foot-print of the animal which the soul of the departed will inhabit in next life.

Witchcraft: The intense hatred of the Gond for witchcraft in which he is a firm believer, is mainly due to the fact that he conceives of it as the unlawful propitiation of supernatural powers, who are enemies of the village and of the racial gods to induce them to bring evil on members of the tribe. When a person is suspected of witchcraft—the victim is usually a woman—she is taken to the nearest stream or pool, in which three men stand. The woman is immersed in the pool while the first man throws an arrow on the second who gathers it and throws it on the third who throws it to the bank. If the woman remains under water while this is being done, she is innocent, if she comes up she is a witch. Her head is shaved, her front teeth knocked out and she is banished from the village.

ETHNO-MEDICAL BELIEFS

The health culture of the tribal population upholds three categories of ethnomedical therapy based on indigenous health tradition and community belief system. These therapeutic procedures are herbal or chemotherapy, mechanical therapy and magico-religious therapy. Under chemotherapy, an indigenous heating method is administered to draw medicinal extracts from herbs and organs of the animals, whereas strict observation of traditional rituals along with chanting of mantras generating sound vibration by Shamans are prescribed to invoke grace and favour of supernatural forces in curing the diseases under magico-religions therapy. The indigenous therapeutic procedures administered for the use of medicated oils, medicinal herbs, medicinal extracts from animals, for treatment of bone setting, branding, blood letting to eliminate disorder in human system and rectify biological dysfunction of the human body are categorised as mechanical procedures. These therapeutic procedures are very complex and interwoven in the ethnomedical culture of tribals in Chhattisgarh as well as other forest regions in India.

The causes of diseases are attributed to supernatural and natural or physical factors supported by traditional values and folk belief system. Their knowledge and belief regarding the origin, causes and treatment of diseases differs from that of the modern medical health system. They therefore depend more on the folk healing system, which holds symbolic and more meaningful significance for their community. They strongly attribute supernatural factors such as soul loss spirit intrusion, spirit of sickness, breach of taboo as the causes of human diseases, which are specifically diagnosed by Baiga or Shamans who are experts in magico-religions healing. They believe that evil spirits causing diseases dwell in graveyards, on cremation grounds, in old tamarind trees and in abandoned places. The sacrifice of a fowl, along with the offering of liquor and the performance of rituals, invites pleasure and satisfaction of these spirits, who leave the body of patients without torturing them.

The human factors contributing to the prevalence of diseases are classified as evil eye, evil touch, evil mouth and sorcery. Under natural factors, the objects carrying diseases and intrusion, including treatment by modern medical professionals, are considered negative elements, violating the values of ethno-healing practices and the traditional belief system. These are considered negative forces that promote diseases in the human world.

(a) Reproduction System—Menstruation and Menopause

When a woman is in her menstrual period, she stays apart and may not cook for herself nor touch anybody nor sleep on a bed made of cotton thread. The Gonds have a separate house outside the village to which women have to retire at this time. When a woman is with child for the first time her women friends come and give her green clothes and bangles; they then put her into a swing and sing songs. While she is pregnant she is made to work in the house so as not to be inactive. If the birth is delayed they put a few grains of gram into the woman's hand and then some one takes and feeds them to a mare, as it is thought that the woman's pregnancy has been prolonged by her having walked behind the tethering-ropes of a mare, which is twelve months in foal. Or she is given water to drink in which a Sulaimani bead or a rupee of Akbar's time has been washed.

Chickenchura is a powder that is given to a woman suffering from white discharge.

(b) Pregnancy Stages

The Gonds believe that the baby becomes able and capable of moving into the womb exactly after the completion of four and a half months period of gestation and is able to rotate in the womb till the completion of 7 months. Further from month 7 to 9, the baby grows with a fastest pace and is ready for delivery by the end of 9th month.

A pregnant woman must not look on a dead body or her child may be still-born and she must not see an eclipse or the child may be born maimed. Women of the Mang, Mahar, Gond and Dhimar castes act as midwives. Sometimes when delivery is delayed they take a folded flower and place it in a pot of water and believe that as its petals unfold so the womb will be opened and the child born, or they seat her on a wooden bench and pour oil on her head, her forehead being afterwards rubbed with it, in the belief that as the oil falls so the child will be born.

(c) Delivery

In case of swelling on the legs (eclampsia/hypertension), the mother is given mashed bananas as it helps in reduction of this swelling. In case the mother is not able to deliver the child then her husband is asked to go to the community well, fetch a bucket of water just with one hand and then this water is given to the mother three times after regular intervals, and then the delivery takes place. The belief is that this water provides energy to her to deliver the baby and helps in *nazar utarna*.

After the delivery, the father is considered to be impure for one month and does not go out for work for one entire month. The father may reap the crop, but cannot thresh or sow till the umbilical cord of the child drops of. Between the fifth and twelfth day after the borth the mother is purified and the child is named. On this day, the child's hair is shaved by the son-in-law of the family or the brother-in-law of the father or mother.

(d) Treatment of Umbilical Cord

The umbilical cord is cut by the lady who conducts the delivery and then the cord is buried in the ground, fire is set on this place, the land is burnt and then it is covered with mud.

(e) Breast Feeding

The Gonds believe that during child birth, the mother loses all her energy and heat and hence her body turns cold. The perception is that coldness of body can also lead to unconsciousness, filling of air in the brain, which might lead to mental abnormality. So, there is a need to generate heat in her body and for this purpose special diet is given, this comprises of Kurta dal, Saunth and Ajwain, many times the saunth and ajwain are mixed in wheat and are given in form of chapattis. The generation of body heat is extremely important as that ensures circulation of blood and production of breast milk. The Gonds also feel that apart from this food, the mother is just given kheer made out of milk for the first five days, as consumption of other food items might dilute the colostrum milk, which may not be good for the baby. This importance of colostrum milk is understood well and essentially given to the baby.

The practice of breastfeeding is very common and is maintained for a long period. The smooth secretion of breastmilk among anaemic lactating women poses a serious problem for sustaining breastfeeding practices for the survival of neonates. This adds to the increase in neonatal and infant mortality in these communities. The milk of the tigress mixed with rice or bread has been administered under the guidance of Shamans as medicinal dosage for enhancing breastmilk among breastfeeding mothers. One dose is enough to rectify this reproductive health deficiency.

TRADITIONAL BIRTH CONTROL PRACTICES

The Gonds are fully aware that certain diseases have a natural cause, and they know many jungle medicines to cure such diseases. But when these remedies remain ineffective, they resort to magical devices.

The Understanding About Disease

The diagnosis of diseases by the Gond tribe of Naoradehi is interesting because they live in interior, inaccessible area and lack the use of modern scientific equipment's for treatment. They do not express the exact causes behind the disorders however, using their eyes, ear, nose and hand they can check a base and tell the treatment of diseases.

They believe that all ailments as caused by supernatural forces and the Patel (headmen) is the only hope for curing all ailments. It is observed among Gond tribal community that one man is not knowledgeable about the treatment of all diseases. However, they treat diseases by medicinal plants.

Traditional Healers

The Bhumak or Pujari is usually a Gond or Dhimar. He receives the same dues from the cultivators as the Garpagari. His business is to perform the customary worship of the village deities at the prinicipal festivals, and to attend on and provide for the wants of Government officials, who visit the village. On a Sunday or Wednesday in May the Bhumak performs the Bidri Puja, at which offerings subscribed for by the cultivators are made to all the village gods for the success of the crop. He offers some seed rice to the gods, placing it on a mango leaf, and then takes it all round the village, giving a few grains to each cultivator, who mixes them with his seed-grain and thereafter commences sowing.

Many villagers have also a Bhagat or priest of Devi, who is a Gowari or Dhimar. The qualification for being a Bhagat is to be possessed by the deity, in which case the gifts of divination and prophecy are held to accrue. The present Bhagat of the Bondgaon Devi is a local celebrity and makes progresses through the District followed by a train of as many as fifty persons. When he comes to a village the people assemble and he makes prophecies, telling those whose relatives are sick whether they will recover, or whether they will obtain property which has been lost or stolen, and so on. Other Bhagats make a little hut in front of Devi's shrine and place a flag on it, and from here they give oracles to those who come to consult them. The method of divination by swinging a lamp is also much practised, the answer being in the affirmative or negative according to the direction in which the lamp swings. The lamp in suspended from a stick by a sling made of human hair or of somebody's cast off sacred thread. If a man wishes to make inquiry about some other person from the Bhagat, he takes a handful of rice and carries it round him, and then takes and places it before the Bhagat, to represent the other person. If a man is bitten by a snake, the Bhagat comes and draws water from a well, and, muttering some charm, gives it to the patient to drink; he will then recover and the symptoms of snake-poisoning will appear in the Bhagat for an hour or two.

To Avoid Pregnancy

In order to avoid pregnancy special diet is given to the mother after the delivery who does not want to have child immediately. The diet specifically consists of jaggery and sesame seeds cooked up together in the form of small cakes or balls. This helps in not only avoid immediate conception as they believe that both the items generate extreme heat, the conception is avoided, plus it also helps her in gaining overall energy in her body.

Abortion Techniques

The banana root is dipped in Navsagar and then inserted into the vagina, in next 24 hours or so there is heavy bleeding and this also causes abortion of the baby, this is done immediately after it is identified that the woman has missed her period and has not been having menstruation for almost one and a half to two months.

Omdas Tirgude is the local healer from Parastola village in Gondia, and he prepares tablets made out of wheat and Dhatura tree, which, consumed by the pregnant woman in the early days of pregnancy, especially first one and half months would lead to abortion. To stop bleeding he knows a mantra and he visits the mother who has just delivered recites the mantra.

Rahul Ramaji Ramteke is a Vaidu from Parastola, he is a literate and refers to a book that was written in 1847 by Dr. Aina Puri Shastri, which has been published by a publisher from Mumbai and is in Hindi language.

He prescribes a traditional contraceptive to women of the village, this entails a mixture of Neem, Awla and Beheda, which according to him is a combination of hot and cold plant elements which is given to the women on 5th day of their menses, every third month in order to avoid conception. Plant materials like raw papaya, kapas seed, parathi pala (green grass), kate korati (root) and hirakasi (root) is used for avoiding conception.

Gonds apply *Gloriosa superba - rhizome* (Kalihari, Kathari, Kulhari, Languli) extract over the navel and vagina. It induces labour pain and performs normal delivery. Bhumkas (local healers) generally prescribe 250 to 500 mg of the rhizome as dosage. According to Bhumkas of Patalkot, this dose may lead to abortion if given to a lady with pregnancy of 1 or 2 months. Since the rhizome is having abortive action, this is prescribed for normal delivery.

In Ayurveda and Yunani systems of medicine, the tuber of plant is well known due to its pungent, bitter, acrid, heating, anthemintic, laxative, alexiteric and abortifacient nature. It is widely used in the treatment of ulcers, leprosy, piles, inflammations, abdominal pains, intestinal worms, thirst, bruises, infertility and skin problem. However, ingestion of all parts of the plants is extremely poisonous and can be fatal. *Gloriosa superba* is mixed with ghee and used orally in order to induce abortion.

To induce and accelerate delivery

When the woman is unable to get the labour pains and is not able to deliver the child, a root called Kanukilla is kept in her hair, this accelerates the delivery process.

To Ensure Conception

Tender leaves of banyan tree are mixed with the material that comes out while the monkey is delivering the placenta.

This mixture is given to women every second month and this helps the woman in conceiving the child.

For Treating Impotency and Arousing Sexual Desire

A lot of problems related to infertility are directly linked with the fact that the man or the woman can be impotent and hence a lot of herbs are used by Gonds to treat impotency and this factor is considered very important for every married couple.

Following are the herbs used for the treatment as well as to arouse sexual desire:

- Butea monosperma (Lamk.) Taub. Syn. Butea frondosa Koen. ex. Roxb.
  Family: Papilionaceae
  Local Name: Palas
- Ricinus communis Linn.
  Family: Euphorbiaceae
  Local Name: Arandi
- Allium sativum Linn.
  Family: Liliaceae
  Local Name: Lahsun
- Carica papaya Linn.
  Family: Caricaceae
  Local Name: Papeeta
- Euphorbia hirta Linn.
  Family: Euphorbiaceae
  Local Name: Dudhi
- Trigonella foenum-graecum Linn.
  Family: Leguminosae
  Local Name: Methi
- Bryonia laciniosa Linn.
  Family: Cucurbitaceae
  Local Name: Shivlingi
- Ficus religious Linn.
  Family: Moraceae
  Local Name: Papal

- Hibiscus rosa-sinensis Linn.
  Family: Malvaceae
  Local Name: Jason, Gurhal
- Mangifera indica L.
  Family: Anacardiaceae
  Local Name: Aam
- Mucuna prurita Hook. Syn. M. pruriens (L.) DC. Local name: Kimaach Family: Papilionaceae .

7

Maternal Health and Birth Control Practices of the Mavchi Tribe

PROFILE OF MAVCHIS

According to the Census of India population of Mavchi tribe is not given because this tribe is not distinctly found in the Constitutional list of tribals in the State of Maharashtra. Given below is decadel population of Gamit/Gamta.

Population

The decadel growth of the population of Gavit or Gamta as per the Census of India is given in Table 7.1.

Table 7.1

Decadel Growth of Gamit population

Sr. No.	*Year*	*Total population*
1.	1961	102,321
2.	1971	128,831
3.	1981	110,828
4.	1991	122,407

Source: Census of India

Origin of Mavchis: Diverse Opinions

According to R.E.Enthoven (1920) the Gamits have synonyms like Gamta, Gavit, Mavchi and Padvi. Gamit means a villager. In Gujarat Mavchis are known as Gamits, Gamta and Gavits. In Gujarat, they are chiefly distributed in the hilly terrains and on the plains of Surat, Valsad, Dang and Bharuch district. According to the 1981 census, their population in Gujarat including the Gamta, Gavit, Mavchi and Padvi is 250,837.

R.E. Enthoven (1920) is of the opinion that the Gamits/ Mavchis migrated to Maharashtra and Gujarat from their original home in Goa. According to K.S. Singh (1998) the Gavits believe that their ancestors were warriors in Rana Pratap's army and that they migrated to the present habitat in the course of war.

Clans

Some of the popular clans of Mavchi tribe are Mavchi, Gavit, Thingle, Mavali, Choudhari, Kuwar, Barish, Raut, Desai, Bhavre, Bilkude etc. Marriage within the clan is prohibited.

Geographical Distribution

The members of Mavchi tribe are found principally in Nawapur and Sakri tahsils of Nandurbar district in the State of Maharashtra. Distribution of Mavchi tribe in Nawapur tahsil. They are found in following villages.

1. Kareghat
2. Khokarwada
3. Lakkadkot
4. Zamanjat
5. Khekda
6. Thuva
7. Ampada
8. Gadad
9. Bhavar
10. Bandarphali
11. Karanji Khurd

12. Bhil Manjre
13. Ahirvihir
14. Raipur
15. Pralapur
16. Vad Kalambi
17. Nagzari
18. Khoksa
19. Ghamor
20. Kor Khamb
21. Borpada
22. Karanji Budruk
23. Bolipada
24. Gatadi
25. Dapur
26. Mohanpada
27. Pipran
28. Rayangan
29. Chinchpada
30. Visarwadi Mothi
31. Lahan Vvisarwadi
32. Wakipada
33. Nawapur

Distribution of Mavchis in Sakri tahsil

1. Varthali
2. Bipkhel
3. Rampura
4. Umaryamal

5. Manjri
6. Shendwal
7. Pimpalpada
8. Chokhad
9. Daskhel
10. Lakhane
11. Kalamba
12. Varsa
13. Shiladi
14. Malgaon
15. Khirgaon
16. Malamba
17. Bandharpale
18. Parsari
19. Daripas
20. Khair Khunda
21. Ambur
22. Busraval
23. Umberpath
24. Madalipada
25. Ketak
26. Keli
27. Gavali
28. Choranmala
29. Chopale
30. Sakri

The Mavchis also called as Gamta, Gavits in South Gujarat region are concentrated in Vyara, Songadh and Valod tahsils of Surat district, wherein they constitute on overwhelming majority of population. While some of them are found in Dharampur, Vansada, Valia, Sagbara and Dediapada (Satyakam Joshi 2000: 268)

Physical Features

According to Karve and Dandekar (1951) the Mavchis are mostly short or below medium in stature and have broad faces with a flat nose and show mesocephalic features. According to Vyas et.al (1958), they indicate a high incidence of gene A and presence of A_2 allele in a very low value (1 per cent). They also show a relatively higher proportion of gene N (46 per cent) in the M.N. blood group system, than do other proto-Australoid groups of Central India.

Dress Pattern

The Mavchi men wear dhoti (*Favya*) and Shirt. Some men wear turban called pagdi, while others prefer white Nehru cap. The women wear sari called *lugde* and blouse. Half a piece of the sari cloth is used to cover their head and the body. Women folk are known to wear bright and colourful saris. The spinsters of Mavchi community wear blouse (*dhovi*) and sari (*lugdi*). A girl who attains puberty starts wearing sari and blouse. Infact, that is a signal for eligible batchlors, that she is due for marriage.

Ornaments

Mavchi women like the Bhil and Pawra women are very fond of ornaments. Elderly women and widows wear white bead necklaces.

Family Type

Nuclear families are very common among the Mavchis, however few cases of joint families too are observed. Patriarchy, patrilinyh and patrilocal residency by cultural rules are the family forms.

Kinship Terminology

The kinship terminology as observed among the Mavchis from an emic perspective as found in their Mavchi dialect is given below:

Sr. No.	*Kinship term in English*	*Kinship term in Mavchi dialect*
1.	Father	Abo
2.	Mother	Ayo
3.	Brother	Baha
4.	Sister	Bahi
5.	Grand Father	Abaho Doho
6.	Grand Mother	Ajeehee
7.	Paternal Uncle	Phuyo
8.	Paternal Aunt	Phuheeo
9.	Maternal Uncle	Maamaho
10.	Maternal Aunt	Phuyee
11.	Sister-in-law	Halee
12.	Brother-in-law	Haalaho
13.	Father-in-law	Haahyeho
14.	Mother-in-law	Hahoo
15.	Son-in-law	Jaavahaan
16.	Daughter-in-law	Bahoo
17.	Grand Son	Naatanay
18.	Grand Daughter	Naatanee
19.	Father's brother's son	Phuye Poho
20.	Father's brother's daughter	Phuye Pohi
21.	Mother's brother's son	Mamuna Poyarya
22.	Mother's brother's daughter	Bohee
23.	Mother's sister's son	Bhasa
24.	Mother's sister's daughter	Phuyee Hobi
25.	Father's eldest brother	Abo Modo Paahoo
26.	Mother's eldest sister	Ayo Modo Bohi
27.	Son-in-law's father	Javaahee Abo

(Contd...)

Sr. No.	*Kinship term in English*	*Kinship term in Mavchi dialect*
28.	Son-in-law's mother	Javaahee Ayo
29.	Elder sister	Mothi Bohi
30.	Elder brother	Motho Baha
31.	Youngest sister	Chhoto Bohi
32.	Youngest brother	Chhoto Baha
33.	Great Grandfather	Mothaa Abaa
34.	Great Grandmother	Mothi Ajeehee
35.	Sister's son	Bhasoo
36.	Step Mother	Jeejeehee
37.	Parents	Aaeeho Aabaho
38.	Father's younger brother	Dihoo
39.	Wife	Thaie
40.	Husband	Mati
41.	Forefathers	Wadvadil
42.	Twins	Judvo Poyarya
43.	Sister's son	Panjah
44.	Sister's daughter	Paanjeehee

Forms of Marriage

Monogamy is common among the Mavchis, however one gets to rarely see few cases of polygamy. The Mavchis do not permit polyandry. Marriage by capture was prevalent among the Mavchis once, is slowly dying off as quite a few of them have taken up Christianity. The elderly people in the tribe manage marriages.

A Mavchi boy chooses and decides the girl to whom he has to marry. He informs about his fiance to his parents. The parents along with 10 to 15 elders from the boy's village go to visit the girl's family. They discuss in detail about the relationship. The bride's consent is taken. The girl's parents along with few elders offer "*Manha*", the traditional wine prepared from the flowers of *Madhuca indica*. The bride's parents some times offer food to the groom's party. After 8 to 10 days, the groom's people revisit the bride's village to pay the Bride price.

Traditionally bride price (*dej*) was given in kind. We asked several old men to find how much bride price had they given. Most of them said 2 to 5 bags of Jawar and between Rs. 11/- to Rs. 501/-. The latest sum is either Rs. 550/- or 555/-. Besides this amount, the groom has to take care of expenses of food, clothes, ornaments and liquor. It is only after giving the bride price the date of wedding is fixed.

On the day of wedding the groom's party goes to the bride's village in a procession accompanied by a musical band. The groom's brother leads the procession. He carries a pot of foodgrains brought from the groom's home. The pot or the bag, which contains these grains, is called "*Joda*" in Mavchi dialect. This bag or pot is given to the bride's father on reaching the village. The action of accepting foodgrains by the bride's father symbolises permission given by him and his villagers for the wedding ritual. Yet another ritual performed during the wedding by the Mavchis is the "turmeric application ritual". The bride and the groom are applied turmeric on the face, hands and legs and given bath ritually in the presence of family members, relatives and the tribesmen.

This ritual is performed one day prior to the wedding. Both the parties exchange turmeric as well as liquor. Pendols (Mandaps) are errected seperately in front of the houses of the bride and the groom. The exchange of liquor and turmeric symbolises the bond between both the families.

The person who presides over the wedding ritual is "Punjari" , a priest of the tribe. He performs the wedding. The traditional pendol (mandap) errected in front of the house of the bride as well as the groom is a squarish erection made up of branches of ficus glomerata (*Umbar*). This is also decorated by the leaves of *Palas* (Butea frondosa) and *Jamun* (Elegenia Jombolina). In this pendol, the turmeric ceremony as well as the main wedding ritual takes place.

The groom's sister and her husband get the honour of applying turmeric to the groom first. Yet another custom is of moving around "Darwaza" the central pillar of the house nine times in an anti-clock fashion, by the couple. The Mavchis respect this pillar and believe that the house of the Mavchis rest on this sole pillar.

After this the couple is carried on the shoulders of close relatives in a musical procession, to a tree called, *"Hengala"* while others drink and dance, The Punjari (Priest) makes the couple to hold the leaves of the tree and declares them as husband and wife. The speciality of this tree is that its leaves are naturally one such that these look these two as well as one. The Mavchis believe that a couple, after marriage should be "one" like these leaves although they look two.

The guests who come for the wedding are given "Mauha liquor" and food. The food is usually dal (pulse) and rice. After the food, the groom and the bride exchange rings (*Mundi*) of silver. The groom also gives a silver chain to the bride. The visitors offer gifts to the newly wedded couple called *"Aher"*. This usually consists of utensils and items of utility.

Musical instruments such as *Pawri* (wind instrument), *Dhol* (drum), *Sanj* (cymbals) are played before and after the wedding. Every one attending the wedding drinks and dances.

An old woman called *"Path rakhin"* (escort) is sent to the boy's house for a period of nine days. She permits them to sleep together. The groom's people give *"Pathrakhin"* gifts such as sari, blouse, towel and/or ornaments, depending on the economic condition of the groom's family.

According to K.S. Singh (1998: 134-135) "the Mavchi are divided into a few flans (*atak*) which no longer regulate their marriage alliances. Now-a-days while arranging a marriage alliance, they avoid only close relations. At present, Gavit is used a surname by all of them. The Mavchi consider the Vasave, Tadvi, Valvi and Naik as communities of equal status with whom marriage alliances are possible. Consonguineous marriages are preferred with the mother's brother's daughter or with the father's sister's daughter. Marriage through negotiation and by service, intrusion, capture and elopment are the common modes of acquiring spouses. Negotiation, however is the most popular form. Polygamy, Junior Sororate and Junior levirates are allowed in this community. Bride price is paid. Generally, the boys get married between eighteen to twenty years of age and the girls by the age of sixteen. Divorce is permitted and widow re-marriage is allowed. A decrease in the frequency of marriage by service, polygamy an increase in the amount of bride price, wearing of a necklace and applying vermilion mark as symbols of marriage for women are the social changes that have taken place recently. Residence after marriage is patrilocal though a few cases of matrilocal residence also exist.

Delivery Ritual

The first delivery takes place at the bride's parent's home. During the eight month of pregnancy, the bride is sent to her parent's house for first delivery. The delivery takes place at home. The traditional Birth Attendant called, "*Huvarki*" or "*Dain*" performs the delivery. The parents give her Rs. 5/- to Rs. 50/-, food grains, clothes and/or liquor for her services.

Panchvi Pujan (*Pachraha*)

On the fifth day, "*Pachraha*" the "*Huvarki*" the Traditional Birth Attendent performs ritual. The naming ceremony of the newborn takes place, after which close relatives and friends are given food and "*Mauha-Horo*" liquor.

Religion

Animism is a typical feature of the Mavchi religion. Every Mavchi village has a "gram dev" village god situated on the northern side of the village. Some of the principal deities of the Mavchis are Monger (crocodile), Waghdev, Kakadeha and Mandar dev. According to K.S.Singh (1998), the main village deity is Daman Devi, which is worshipped during Dussehra. Some of them worship Hanuman as well . The *Mandar* (goval dev) and the village deity is worshipped one week before holi festival. The Christian Mavchis go to church and believe in Christ, at the same time continue with their traditional cultural rituals. These gods are offered liquor, eggs, rice, goat, chicken and coconut and worshipped. The blood of the goat/chicken is sprinkled on the idol of the village god.

Khamb—The Acenstral Memorial

The Mavchis bury their dead. An ancestral memorial of wood is errected on the tomb. This wooden pillar is called Khamb. Lately they have started making images of a man and or woman depending on the sex of the deceased.

According to K.S.Singh (1998: 135) the Mavchi bury the dead along with the personal belonging of the deceased.

A dead pregnant woman's foetus is removed and burried seperately. Memorial stones, known as "Khatra" are errected in the memory of the brave and old persons.

Burial Practice

Whenever there is death in Mavchis, every home donates Rs. 5 to support the greaved family. This money is used for the expenses of the burial service. The dead person is laid on a wooden cot. There is a person in the Mavchi village called *shravaniya* who is responsible for conducting the burial service. The dead body is carried on shoulders, till the village boundary. At the village boundary the body is lowered down for a while and the women return home. Women are not allowed to visit the burial ground. *Shravanya* walks in front of the body holding an axe, upside down. While walking he drops rice grain on the ground. After reaching the burial ground, the body is lowered in the burial pit.

Seven rounds of the body are made near the pit, and then the body is lowered into the pit. The food is kept near the pit. They believe that the dead will eat that food. *Shravaniya* lays his hand on the relative of the dead person, to bless him for offering food to the dead person. After this, *shravaniya* puts mud into the pit and others follow him until the pit is fully covered with mud. Before returning home they wash themselves in the river water nearby. When a person dies in accident or a murder case then, they make a statue of that person and keep that at the place where the dead body is buried. The place is such, which can be noticed from far away place of the village. It is on the roadside. But those who die after sickness or naturally, for them they make a tomb like a house on it. They believe that the spirit of the dead person should not come to their homes and disturb them. The spirit should stay in that house.

Traditional Political System

A council of village elders manage village/hamlet level affairs. This organisation works on certain laws. Disputes over land, divorce, seperation, quarrels etc. are solved by the council of village elders. Key personnel such as Punjari (Priest), medical practitioners, village head etc. play significant role in maintaining the integrity of the traditional political system.

Festivals

The main festival of Mavchi is *Waghdev* (Tiger god). It is observed in the month of August every year. This festival is observed to please Tigers who used to destroy human being as well as animals. The branch of the Teakwood is placed in the middle of the land considering it as Tiger God. Buffalo or goat is offered to this god and the community take part in community food cooked near the river. Along with this other Hindu festivals are also celebrated.

According to Satyakam Joshi (2000: 269) the most important festivals of the Gamits are Diwali, Holi, Balev and Gamdev. Diwali is considered to be an important festival. First day after Diwali is known as Gamdev (festival of village god). Villagers gather at one place and worship the Gamdev. Young boys and girls dance on that day.

Holi festival lasts for about twenty days. During Holi, Gamit dance in-groups with their traditional musical instruments like Doharu, Dhol, Tur, Kundi etc. In addition, there are other festivals associated with sowing and harvesting of crops, wherein godess Kansari is worshipped. The Nandario dev festival marks the beginning of rainy season. Some of these festivals appear to be dying out. This is especially the case with Holi and Diwali in South Gujarat.

Music and Dance Forms

The Mavchi tribe uses the following musical instruments:

(a) *Pawri:* "Pawri" is a wind musical instrument like that of the "*Tarpa*" of the Warlis. Pawri is made up of a dry gourd, which is about 2 feet long. Flute like hollow bamboo sticks are attached in it with the help of honey comb wax. The bamboo sticks are six-inch long with 3 holes on each. Towards the end of these sticks a saxophone like lower part is attatched. This part is made up of spathe of the phoenix sylvester (palm). It is bound with the help of the wax. The difference between Tarpa and Pawri is that, the Tarpa is played by blowing air from the apex of the instrument while Pawri is played from the side, i.e. by blowing air in the middle of the longish gourd.

Pawri by traditional cultural norms of the Mavchi is played by male only. Females are not allowed to play Pawri. This is true among the Warlis too. Warli women are not allowed to play Tarpa.

(b) *Dhol:* A Dhol is a drum, the circular body of which is made up of teak or ain tree. Skin of a bull, cow or goat is used on either sides of the circular structure. Dhol too is played by a male member of the tribe.

(c) *Jhangli:* A Jhangli is a string instrument like the "*ghangli*" of the Warlis. It is made up of two oval or round dry gourds, which are attatched by a bamboo on which two strings are tied. The strings are tighthened with the help of a bamboo bridge which rests on the stick.

Dance Forms

The Mavchis have two dance forms namely:

Pawri Dance: This dance is performed using the Pawri, which is played by a male Mavchi. Nearly 50 to 150 males and females dance to the tune of this instrument. This dance is performed during Holi and Diwali.

Chibali Dance: Chibali is a basket which is decorated with coloured ribbons and wollen threads. Mavchi women hold this basket on the head and perform this dance during weddings.

RITUALS OF TRANSITION

What is a ritual?

The term 'ritual' though seems to be a simple matter, few terms in the study of religion have been explained in more confusing ways. For example, Edmund Leach (1968:524) a cultural anthropologist after noting the general disagreement among the anthropological theorists, suggests that the term 'ritual' should be applied to all the cultural sets of behaviour, that is the symbolic dimension of human behaviour as such regardless of its explicit religious, social or other content.

According to David Lotz (1987:405), a ritual is referred to as those conscious and voluntary repetitions and stylised bodily actions, that are centred on cosmic structures or sacred presence, he includes verbal behaviour such as chants, songs, and prayers in the category of bodity actions. Kartz and Kirkland (1988: 179) are of the view that 'Rituals are stylised, repetitive, arbitary and exaggerated forms of behaviour.'

Turner (1967) uses the term ritual to 'prescribe formal behaviour for occasions not given over to technological routine, having reference to beliefs in mystical (non-empirical) beings or power.'

Rituals are thus a set of stylised bodily actions (which may include iconic symbols such as acts, objects, words, gestures, prayers, songs, chants and other things) performed in a culturally defined place, situation or context by certain actor/s only, encompassing basic rules to accomplish given tasks or goals in any social sphere within a given cultural frame of reference.

A number of social scientists interested in socio-cultural functions of rituals in different spheres of life have pointed out varied functions of rituals which are as follows:

- Rituals encourage cohesion (Gluckman 1970)
- Rituals facilitate transition (Van Gennep 1960)

- Rituals define conceptual categories (Mary Douglas 1966)
- Enhance individual and group autonomy (Kartz P. 1981)
- Help resolve social conflicts (Gluckman 1970; Turner 1967)
- Endow culturally important cosmological conceptions and values with persuasive emotive force, thus unifying individual participants into a genuine community (Geertz and Turner)
- Ritual actions express and communicate shared socio-cultural meanings which are symbolically transacted through the medium of ritual action (Munn 1973)
- They reveal the knowledge of meanings of symbols involved in them (Hongiman 1959)
- They are modes of symbolic communication (Firth 1973)

From the theoretical understanding it is observed that rituals are set of culturally governed symbolic activities, which gain meaning with in a given context, situation or culturally defined place and that these rituals reveal socio-cultural concepts of the natives and are performed to accomplish tasks or goals in any social sphere.

Given this background, the rituals of transition of the Mavchi Tribe right from birth to death are presented in this chapter.

Pregnancy Rituals

Mavchis do not observe any pregnancy rituals. Pregnant women however take the advice of the *Huvaki* – the Traditional Birth Attendant regarding any problem associated with pregnancy .

Birth Ritual

Delivery by the *Huvaki* is conducted in the kitchen. The head of the delivery woman is always towards the east. The unbelical cord is buried in the manger towards the eastern side. The Mavchis do not differentiate between the male and female child.

Pachraha Ritual

On the fifth day after the delivery of the Mavchis celebrate the *Pachraha* ritual. The *Huvaki* worships the pounding hole – a symbol of earth's sex organ. She puts nine heaps of rice on the eastern side of the "*Ukali*" the pounding hole. The midwife gets Rs. 5/- as her fees for delivering the new born. The fees has now risen upto Rs. 200/-. The Mavchi people celebrate this ritual by giving food to the near and dear ones.

The ritual of *Pachraha* is symbolic of the Mavchi perception about fertility. The *ukali* symbolises the sex organ of the earth, while the *pounder* symbolises sex organ of the sun. Pachraha ritual symbolises sexual union of the sun and earth.

Marriage Ritual

Monogamy is the most popular form of marriage, however polygamy is permitted. Marriage by capture is socially sanctioned. A Mavchi boy who likes a Mavchi girl is socially permitted to pick up the girl from a village market and bring her home. The negotiations take place later on. Arranged marriage is the principal norm though prominent among the marriage rituals are :

Olada Chadva: Application of turmeric to the groom and the bride by their family members in their respective homes, on the first day.

Orad Lavana: Actual wedding ritual performed near the "*Hingla*" (Bauhinia ricimosa tree) on the second day in the bride's village.

Olada Utada: The removing of turmeric from the body of the bride on the third day of the wedding.

Bride Price: The Mavchi term for bride price is "*Jogda*". The groom's people pay something in cash and kind to the bride's parents. When Surnya an old man from Rayangan village, got married 60 years ago he paid Rs. 20/- and 15 Kg. Rice as bride price.

Death Ritual

Among the Mavchis they bury their dead. Their graveyards are usually situated towards the south of the village. They bathe the dead body and put on clean clothes. The clothes worn are buried along with the body. The death ritual is performed by a Shaman called "*Saravanya*". The head of the body's head always points the south. The belonging of the dead are buried with the body.

Soul Migration Ritual

On the 12th day after the death the Mavchis conduct the "*Barmoha* Ritual". This ritual is presided over by the "*Sarnya*". He puts food on four corners of the grave. The food carried in a colourless "*Chhibali*" – death basket, without any decoration. A widow burries her ornaments given by her husband during wedding in his grave. Some women keep it in the house in a box or "*bodhadi*" – the grain basket.

The *Khamb*: Ancestral Memorial

Different types of ancestral memorial called *Khamb* are erected on the grave of the dead. These are prepared by a caste group called "*Takara*". Each pillar costs Rs. 800-900.

The natural life cycle goes on as life moves.

The Epidemic Ritual

In times of epidemics every Mavchi family sweeps dust and garbage out of their houses. Put the same in a basket and throw it out on the southern boundary of the village. The garbage in this context symbolises epidemics.

The action of sweeping symbolises removing the epidemic out of the village. Healing Rituals associated with epidemics are prevalent all tribes. Hence the entire community participates health rituals associated with epedemics.

MATERNAL AND CHILD HEALTH CARE BELIEFS AND PRACTICES

The researchers were interested in investigating how traditional beliefs and practices influence the health of mothers and children in the Mavchi tribe of Nawapur tahsil, Dhule district of Maharashtra. They live in small settlements popularly known as "*padas*". Their main occupation is farming. Indebtedness is a common feature among them; they often borrow money for purchase of seeds, cattle, fertilizers and for marriages and other important ceremonies. The tribe has its own religious beliefs. However, although a number of families have been converted to Christianity.

The aims and objectives of the study were:

- To study the food habits of mothers and children;
- To highlight the disease causational concepts of the Mavchis;
- To assess the ritualistic and therapeutic role of traditional medical practitioners with respect too maternal and child health care;
- To explore various rituals and ceremonies associated with puberty, pregnancy, childbirth, marriage and death.

Informants were non-randomly selected from four Mavchi hamlets of the Nawapur tahsil. Indepth interviews with 25 elderly women, two pregnant women and two "*Huvakis*" and a "*Bhagat*" were conducted to gather information associated with maternal and child health care beliefs and practices. The investigators cross-checked this data using participant observation techniques. In addition, they conducted key informant interviews with traditional medical specialists, Primary Health Centre staff and other health care workers.

Food Habits

The Mavchis classify all food items into three categories. Hot foods include items like wheat, brinjal, potato, sunflower oil, papaya, mutton, chicken, gram and other pulses. In addition, the local liquor "*Horo*", prepared from Mahua flowers is considered hot. Cold foods include Sorghum, corn, onion, cabbage, mango, guava, grapes and chickoo. Rice is considered lukewarm, just as various combinations of hot and cold foods are. In cold seasons hot foods are prepared and vice versa. Excessive consumption of hot or cold foods leads to illness, so both the qualities of various foods and their interaction with environmental factors must be taken into account to remain healthy.

While no special diet is prescribed for pregnant women, they should not eat foods that are too hot or too cold, which could adversely affect both the mother and unborn child. For instance, raw papaya is believed to be excessively hot and if eaten by a pregnant woman, may lead to spontaneous abortion. Likewise, pregnant women refuse to take the iron tablets given to them at the public health centre, as these may lead to abortion. Iron tablets were also believed to cause the foetus to grow large, making childbirth difficult.

Solid foods were considered undigestible immediately after delivery. Instead, post delivery new mothers are given "dhasli", a thin rice porridge prepared without salt or sugar, for 15 days. Rice is used instead of corn or sorghum because it is both a lukewarm and a light food. These qualities make it easily digested by the mother and keeps breastmilk lukewarm also, which is beneficial to the child. In addition, "*dhasli*" is believed to increase the production of breastmilk. The porridge must be blend, because salt added to the "*dhasli*" causes swelling in the mother's body and sugar creates heat. When breastmilk is heated due to the sugar intake, it may cause the child to suffer from diarrhoea. To make the "*dhasli*" more palatable, some people prefer to eat it with curd or tur dal. Along the same line, other hot foods like potato, brinjal, chillies and spices, are also avoided after delivery. The Mavchis believe that fish and meat may cause vaginal infection in the mother and sour foods may obstruct the flow of "impure" blood. It is essential that this blood be fully discharged after childbirth.

Mavchi mothers do not breast-feed their newborns for two or three days after delivery. Believed impure, the colostrum is squeezed out and discarded. It is feared that the "thick" and "sticky" nature of this first milk will cause the milk to stick to the lining of the newborn's intestines and prevent the baby from passing the stool. Conversely, as this milk is undigestible, it may lead to diarrhoea or dysentary in the infant. During this period, mothers feed their infants a mixure of honey, cow's milk and water. After the milk comes in, mothers breastfeed their babies for 10-12 months, but not longer. If the breastfeeding period extends for more than one year, the child's teeth will become stained.

Weaning foods are introduced after the fifth month. Solid foods include dal, boiled potato, rice and "*dhasli*". Cow's or goat's milk may be given as a supplementary food before this period, but buffalo milk is avoided until five months, because it is too heavy.

Causes of Illnesses

Illness may be caused by supernatural or natural phenomenon. The Mavchis attribute some illness to the intervention of certain gods, godesses or spirits, or the magical workings of malevolent individuals. Natural causes of illness stem from the lack or excess of such elements as heat, cold, or wind, which upset the bodily balance. Diet and accidents may also be natural causes of ill health.

When illness occurs, it is either ignored, treated with home remedies or referred to a medical specialist. Among the Mavchi tribe four types of medical practitioners are consulted: shamans, bone setters, herbalists, and midwives. The shaman or "*bokta*" is diviner and an interpreter of supernatural phenomena. He is believed to be in direct contact with the spiritual world through the medium of trance. He has one or more spirits at his command. A "*bokta*" provides both psychological and physical relief to his patients by using medicinal herbs and ritual therapy. He may be consulted for ritual purposes, to diagnose and interpret the origin and cause of illness, to administer medicinal herbs, to provide magico-religious therapy, or to ward off the evil spirit or evil eye. Bone setters provide treatment for mechanical injuries such as sprains and broken bones, and use techniques like massage or branding, or apply medicinal herbs. A herbalist is a practitioner who administers herbal medicines. He does not necessarily use magico religious rituals during his treatment. He advises the patients on the correct diet to be followed while ill. The traditional name of the midwife in the Mavchi culture is "*Huvaki*". The "*huvaki*" is always a woman, and not necessarily a diviner. Her duties are to give advice and medical care to expectant mothers, assist in deliveries, and treat illnesses that may befall new mothers and infants. She uses massage techniques, provides dietary advice, and sometimes prescribes herbal medicines.

The following table presents some commonly experienced illness and their origins.

Sr. No.	*Illness*	*Local Name*	*Symptoms*	*Causation*
1.	Measles	Gavaria	Skin turns red marked by blisters and fever	Visitation of goddess
2.	Fever	Joran	Body becomes hot	Possession of exposure to sun
3.	Vomitting	Viti	–	Eating stale food or due to in digestion
4.	Tuberculosis	T.B.	Continuous cough	Drinking local liquor, smoking bidis and chewing tobacco
5.	Leprosy	Kushtrog	Deformity of the nose, fingers and toes	Hereditary
6.	Cough	Khokla	–	Drinking impure water
7.	Leucoderma	Kodla	While patches on body	Hereditary
8.	Scabies	Kharya	Itching, blisters on the skin	Uncleanliness

Important Rituals and Ceremonies

Many of the important rituals in the Mavchi culture are tied to menstruation and childbirth. Menstruation is considered a state of pollution for women; the Mavchis believe that if they consume food prepared by a menstruation woman, it may cause illness. A menstruating woman is therefore socially dislocated from the community. After the menstrual period has stopped, the woman bathes and washes her clothes. She then lights an incence stick, and once again is permitted to interact with others and perform her duties. The purification rite, cleansing her body of evil menstrual blood, places her back into the social system.

The Mavchis believe that the "*atma*" or soul of the child is formed first and later on other bodily parts develop. It takes two and a half months for a girl child and four months for a boy child to develop fully in the womb. During this period the health of the foetus is precarious. A pregnant woman must not interact with an infertile woman; she is a bad omen for both the pregnant woman and her child. During a solar eclipse pregnant woman do not cut vegetables or cook food. They are not allowed to look at the eclipse for fear that the child will be born with a cleft palate or some other congenital deformation.

There is an interesting practice observed during childbirth. The head of the woman in labour should always point to the north, which is considered the direction of life. The "*huvakis*" take care that the woman is not lying in the east-west position, because east symbolises the direction of death. The Mavchis bury their dead with their heads pointing to the east. Another ritual, conducted after childbirth, involves the disposal of the umbilical cord. The cord is buried in the cowshed to prevent it from being used as a magical device by witches and sorcerers to harm the child. After delivery, a woman will not go outside her house for five days. This is to avoid becoming possessed by male evil spirits. Another measure to ward off such spirits is to hang a lemon and five chillies from the door post.

On the fifth day after delivery the naming ceremony takes place, people are invited to attend this auspicious occasion. The midwife has the right to name the child on this day, but the parents may change the name later. "*Horo*", a local liquor prepared from Mahua flowers, is served. The "*huvaki*" takes the first bottle. Men may consume 4-5 bottles each during such an occasion; women 1-2 bottles, and teenage children 1-1/2 bottles. Pregnant woman also drink "*horo*", and during delivery it is compulsory to drink the liquor to forget about the labour pains.

Finally, most prolonged illnesses of infants and children are believed to be the result of the evil eye. To ward off the effect of the evil eye, Mavchis tie a black thread ("*mangadhya*") around the neck of the child. Sometimes yellow and black beads are put around the wrists of infants and children. The black and yellow colors are believed to absorb or neutralise the effect of the evil eye.

Table 7.2

Place of delivery among the Mavchis studied

Sr. No.	*Place of delivery*	*Number*	*Percentage*
1.	Rural hospital	04	4
2.	Primary health center	22	20.05
3.	Home	75	71
4.	Private hospital	04	4
5.	Sub-center	–	–
6.	Others	01	0.5
	Total	**106**	**100**

Table 7.3

Delivery conducted by ANM, doctors and TBAs

Sr. No.	*Conducted by*	*Number*	*Percentage*
1.	ANM	08	7.54
2.	Doctor	02	1.88
3.	TBAs	95	89.62
4.	Others	01	0.94
	Total	**106**	**100**

BIRTH CONTROL PRACTICES

The Mavchis of Nandurbar in the north western part of Maharashtra are geographically distributed in Navapur and Sakri blocks. Majority of Mavchis have become christians. Christian missionaries and medical doctors in Chinchpada Mission Hospital played an important role in imparting family planning and health education to the Mavchis. The influence of christianity and formal education and modernisation did influence the tribe.

Vechya Gavit, a Mavchi resident of Rayangan village, in Navapur tahsil, says about 40 per cent Mavchi educated males and 30 per cent women use modern contraceptives to prevent pregnancies. He also mentioned that Mavchi couples refrain from having sex on the 14th day after the menstrual cycle of a woman. Some couples do not have sex from 12th to 20th day after a woman's periods.

Some of the elderly men from the tribe said that the Mavchi medicine men and TBA's do have knowledge of herbs that prevent pregnancies and induce abortions. The plants mentioned by them were in Mavchi dialect. It is necessary to live with tribals, develop close rapport with elderly people and ethno-medical specialists to explore these plants. Botanists can contribute to great extent to identify the latin name of the herbs used.

THE PROCESS OF DELIVERY

Deliveries among the Mavchis are conducted by T.B.A's called "*Huvarkis*". The *Huvarkis* give advice to pregnant and lactating mothers. When a woman's delivery time is near, she informs elderly women in the family. The *Huvarki* is summoned. The woman is made to lie on the floor and given 2 to 3 pillows or blankets under her head. The *Huvarki* slowly massages the woman's stomach to guide the baby down. She keeps talking to the woman so as to help her conduct normal delivery.

When the baby is out it is wiped with a cloth, then washed with warm water. Its umbilical cord is tied with a cloth. The baby is then given to the mother for breastfeeding.

The Mavchis give colostrum milk to the new born. The T.B.A is given a sari, blouse, liquor and Rs. 100 to 200 these days for conducting delivery. On the fifth day after the delivery she performs the *pachruh* ritual.

COMPLICATIONS

Only very skilled *Huvarkis* are able to handle complicated deliveries because of long years of experience. Still born children are removed by putting hand into the vagina without disturbing the womb. Most Mavchi TBA's refer the complicated cases to Chinchpada hospital or rural hospital at Navapur.

ROLE OF MEDICAL PRACTITIONERS

There are four types of medical practitioners among the Mavchis. They are as follows:

(i) *Shamans (Budwas):* Socio-ritual curers and diviners;

(ii) *Female Shamans (Budvi):* Female socio-ritual curer and diviners;

(iii) *Bone Setters (Had Vaidus):* Who take care of swellings, pains and fractures;

(iv) *Traditional Birth Attendants (Huvarkis):* Who conduct deliveries and give advice to expectant mothers.

All the above medical specialists, including elderly people have wisdom and knowledge about body image, human reproduction birth control practices, medicine ethno-physiology, anatomy etc. and have been the guiding force to their tribesmen for ages.

8

Body Image, Reproduction and Birth Control Practices Among the Ao Nagas

ETHNOGRAPHIC PROFILE OF Ao NAGAS

The Ao tribe is one of the major tribes in the state of Nagaland, occupying the district of Mokokchung. The district is situated in the north-western part of the state. It lies in between 26°10'N - 26°45'N latitudes and 94°15'E and 94°45'E longitude. The district covers an area of 1615 sq km of the total area of the state. Mokokchung town is the headquarter of the district, which is located at an altitude of 1352 m above the sea level.

The district is divided into six different administrative ranges viz, *Asetkong, Changldkong, Japukong, Langpangkong, Ongpangkong* and *Tzurangkong*. According to the census of 2001 (Government of Nagaland 2001), the total population of Mokokchung district is 2,27,230 of which 118,428 is the male population and 1,08,802 is the female population. The rural population constitutes 1,96,026 and urban population is 31,204. The density of population is 142 per sq km. The literacy rate of the district is 84.27 per cent. The male literacy rate is 86.14 per cent and for the female it is 82.20 per cent. The district is characterized by hilly terrain and mountainous area.

The People

The Aos, like their other fellow tribes, are by nature justice loving, self-respecting, fair and sociable people. They are agriculturist by tradition. Rice is their main staple food. Besides agriculture they also practice hunting, fishing and gathering of food and forest products. The day-to-day activities of an Ao Naga villager revolve mainly around shifting cultivation, locally known as *Tekong Lu* and jhum cultivation in the north-eastern India. Both boys and girls begin to work in such fields at the very early age. Their social life centres on festivals, which are mainly agricultural or religious oriented, celebrated with singing, dancing, merry making and feastings marked by wearing of colourful dresses. So far as the Aos traditional, cultural and social life is concerned, all the villages have their own associations and clubs for recreation and socio-cultural and educational welfare.

The etymology of the word' Ao', as held by local traditions and also observed by Mills (1926) is a corruption of the word *'Aor'*, which means 'to go'. [t is said that people who crossed the river Dikhu came to be known as *'Aor';* Dikhu is a river boundary separating the Aos from the Sangtam and the Phom tribes. Thus, *'Aor'* refers to a group of people who went across the river Dikhu.

If one takes a glimpse through the history of the Aos, hardly are there ariy scientific or authentic historical records on their origin. Nevertheless, the only source from which we know much about their origin is drawn from the rich repository of traditions such as legends, myths, and folktales handed down from generations by word of mouth. There is a certain myth that speaks about the origin of the Aos believed to have emerged from *Longterok (long* meaning 'stone' and *terok-'six').* The oral account goes on to say that it was from *Chungliymti* that the Aos crossed the river Dikhu and thence to *Aonglenden;* it was here that ten babies were born. This was the very place where the ten infants were born. Hence the Aos named the place as *Soyim (so-'born', yim-'village').* It was during their stay at *Soyim* that the *Unger* (village chief) was killed by a tiger; thereafter they named the place as *Ungma* (ung-'village chief; *ma-'Iost').* From *Ungma* they proceeded to *Koridang* after which they dispersed to different directions and settled in their respective region. Few cultural materials such as polished stone axes, grinding stones, spindle whorls, pottery vessels, and carnelian beads have been unearthed from *Chungliymti* in recent past by archaeologists (see Nienu 1974, Sharma 1992) that are of great source of historical importance. This set of Neolithic assemblage further lends support to the oral tradition of human occupation of this ancestral settlement.

Another significant position is the close relationship maintained between the Aos and Ahoms. Some vivid accounts also tell us that one of the Queens of the Ahom Raja who was an Ao maiden. In this connection, the Aos and the Ahoms maintained a harmonious matrimonial relationship for a long period of time. In the process, numerous Ao villages received land grants in the plains of Assam in return as gifts and assurance from the Aos to refrain from frequent raids in the plains. With the advent of the British, the relation between the Aos and the Ahoms began to gradually decline but nevertheless they continued to maintain good contacts.

Language

Unlike the other Naga tribes, the Aos comprise of four linguistic groups speaking four different *dialects-Chungli, Mongsen, Changki* and *Sangpur*. Of the four categories, *Mongsen* is considered to be the prototype; while *Chungli* is the official common language owing its roots to the American Baptist Missionaries who first began their activities in a village occupied by the *Chunglirs* and hence introduced their writings in *Chungli*. The fourth *type-Sangpur* was once spoken in the *Sang pur* 'khel' of the *Longsa* village, but is now practically obsolete as reported by Mills (1926). Today, the *Sangpur* speaking group entirely speaks *Chungli*. On the contrary, the *Changki* dialect is akin to the *Mongsen* as it consists of *Mongsen* roots bearing more tonal features. In turn, both these groups share tonal similarities with the Lothas, perhaps as a result of assimilation in the process of migration.

Settlement Pattern

The Ao villages are set up on high summits and steep ridges, which shows a similar pattern with the other Naga tribes. It was important for a village to occupy a site of great focal point for defensive purposes, because of frequent raids with neighbouring villages and between tribes. Several villages still contain the remains of old ditches or moats that were once studded with sharp bamboo spikes, usually poisoned and kept as a trap for the enemies in times of village raids, which is evident from the remains of old village gates now in disuse. The houses around the village are built in more or less continuous fashion, with the main street running along the crest of the ridge and at times built on each side with their front porch facing each other. Moreover, a village is usually surrounded by its land, generally utilised for cultivation purpose, comprising of well defined boundaries with the neighbouring villages. Villages are also commonly found situated close together along the ridges of a range.

House Type

Houses vary from village to village among the Aos. The supporting structures of the house principally consist of wooden posts with the roofs covered with thick thatches of palm leaves or other thatching grass. The porch and backyard are squarish, whereas the ridges of the frontal roof form a tapering gable. The floor and the house walls are chiefly bamboo matted. The traditional division of space inside an Ao house comprises of three compartments: the front of the house usually consists of a miniature room with a beaten mud floor where a pounding table, agricultural implements and domesticated animals are accommodated. This thereafter leads to a large main room that forms the kitchen and the bedroom; further to the backyard, a sitting platform supported by bamboo poles. Except for cane ropes, thatching grass, and bamboos, no other raw materials are employed in such type of traditional structures. Today, these house types have given way to more modern plans with nearly all the houses in the villages built from galvanised roof, wooden planks or cement floorings and brick walls.

Socio-political Organisation

Clans are formed by a group of families who maintain descent from a common ancestor, which may be either patrilineal or matrilineal. Among the Aos, clan membership is strictly patrilineal in character where members of a particular clan are exogamous and any wedlock, if it is to take place, must occur outside a clan. Typical of the Ao clan system is the occurrence of a particular clan not within the confines of a village but also widely dispersed throughout other villages, whereby kinship is traced to a single ancestor. Due to this characteristic, clan bonds are rigid and act as the bottleneck of everyday activities extending from collective efforts of a clan in the construction of its member's house, marriage, agricultural tasks, and also during festive occasions.

The traditional family institution of the Aos is a nuclear unit which must exist independently of any direct parental authority. It is the patriarch custom that determines the male member as the head of this social institution. In the olden days, a male adolescent lived with his parents until he attainted the age of about seven to eight years after which he joined the other boys in the *Ariju* (boy's dormitory). The dormitories or morungs, which is known to the Aos as *Ariju* or the 'educational centre for learning' (Atsongchanger 1995: 14) was not merely a dormitory to sleep in but a learning institution where the young men are taught and trained according to the needs of the village community. However on reaching puberty, a girl may also sleep in the girl's dormitory known as *Zuki* with her female friends (Atsongchanger 1995: 21). It is this *Ariju* institution that played a prominent role in a village where young boys learned their customs and traditions, skills and tactics of warfare, folktales, mythology and all other duties and activities relating to the welfare of the village as well as the individual.

As agriculture is the main stay of the economy, every household in the village are farmers by profession. A traditional exchange system known as barter was prevalent where local commodities such as betel leaves, cotton, chili, ginger, gourds, and mats are taken down to the plains of Assam and traded in exchange for salt and iron. Besides farming, other common professions include blacksmithy, pottery, wood crafts and bamboo matting. But with the impact of education and industrialisation the occupational choices of the people have become more varied, however, options for jobs in governmental sectors outstands the rest.

Traditionally Ao administration is carried out by a council of elders or *Putu Menden* (the word *putu* means 'a generation of thirty years'; *menden-'seat')* where membership to this body is based on clan divisions. Within the membership of the *Putu Menden,* there were certain post-allocations which were also determined on clan divisions. The post of *Ong* (i.e. chief councilor) and the person who holds this post is called the *Onger*. There is only one *Onger* in a *Putu Menden* (Ao, T. 1999: 32). Today the Village Council has taken the place of this body. Likewise is the *Onger,* which has given way to the *Gaonbura* system or the 'Headmen' with the beginning of the British administration.

Also, the institution of *Dobhashi* was introduced by the British to act as interpreters between the locals and the British officials. This was set up so as to adjudicate matters of disputes within villages. In the present day, a village functions under a Village Council that is headed by a Chairman, who is elected by members of the Council; while the members of the Council are nominated by the villagers. The duty of the office is to deal with all important issues relating to the welfare of the village, by way of passing judgment and punishment to the community.

Another important office is the Village Development Board (VDB) set up in 1980-81 in all the State recognised villages (Directorate of Rural Development 2001: ii). Village Development Board looks into the matter of village developmental affairs.

Foraging Behaviour

Besides agriculture, fishing, and hunting-gathering food of forest products are other common daily life activities in a village. Hunting and fishing may be carried out individually, by members of a household, or in groups. Communal hunting is carried out in case of big games like elephant, tiger, bear and wild pigs. Though in the earlier days hunting was carried out with spear, *dao,* blowpipe, and bows and arrows, lately muzzle loading guns are better preferences. Snares are also used to trap games like deer and birds. In addition to hunting, fishing is also carried out with much enthusiasm. All male members of a village take part in such type of expedition known as *Yongok*. Besides hunting and fishing, collection and consumption of variety of wild edible vegetables, roots, stems, ferns, fruits, flowers, mushrooms, and tender shoots of bamboos also constitutes an important diet of the people.

Religion

The traditional religion of the Ao Nagas known as *'Yimsu'* centered around the concept of benevolent and malevolent spirits together with a firm belief on a Supreme God. The propitiation of malevolent spirits is practically the sum and substance of their religion, lest the mysterious power might bring calamities to his door. The Aos believed in one supreme god who is known as *Lijaba AU Yangerba Tsungrem* (Imchen 1993: 78; as opposed to *'Lichaba Ali Yangraba Sangram,'* Majumdar 1925: 21) (meaning 'creator of earth including man and plants'). The use of names of different gods acknowledged by the Ao Nagas is listed as follows (Here the use of the term *Tsungrem* is used in a non-discriminatory way to denote several gods, see Ao, T. 1999: 49):

(a) *Lijaba* is regarded as the creator of the earth and vegetation;

(b) *Lonkitsiingba* is regarded as the God of all heavenly elements and seasons;

(c) *Tiar* or *Tiaba* is regarded as the God of life and death;

(d) *Meyutsiing* or *Mojing* is regarded as the God of truth and justice.

Some of the minor deities recognized by the Aos are *Kini Tsiingrem* (house site deity), *Tekong Tsiingrem* (mountain deity), *Tziiba Tsiingrem* (well deity) and *Along Tsiingrem* (stone deity).

However, with the advent of Christianity in the Ao territory in 1872, spearheaded by Dr. E.N. Clark, mass conversions took place in the region. Interestingly however, deliberate attempts are made by the Ao Christian themselves to identify affinities between Christianity and Ao traditional religion, to argue that the traditional Ao religion provided the basis of foundation for the proclamation of Christianity to the Aos.

Birth Ceremonies

Birth ceremonies played a central role in the family of Ao community. Though sexual discrimination does not exist, sons were favoured. At the time of childbirth, village midwives or generally the mother in-law, attended to all the needs. Pregnant women were guided to proper diet and refrained from carrying heavy loads. Certain food items were impermissible. For instance, pregnant women were not permitted to consume papaya as it may cause miscarriage. Also a peculiar belief during the period of gestation was the taboo to inflict injuries to animals. Even visual contact with animals would lead to the birth of a deformed child, such as resembling the creature they have killed or seen. The presence of the spouse during child birth is important, for it was believed that the unborn baby waits for the father's arrival to the house.

On the third day of the child's birth naming and the ear piercing ceremony is initiated by the father. On this auspicious day, a fowl is killed and the liver fed to the infant. A child is generally named after their grand parents. On the seventh day, the spouses go to the village spring well to bathe. The following day, a fowl and an egg are offered in front of his field house marking the end of the ceremony. Although modern equipments in hospitals and dispensaries around the region have gradually taken the place of traditional ones, there are people who, nevertheless, continue to follow the traditional healing methods predominantly in villages.

Marriage Ceremonies

The Ao marriage system is purely exogamous and marriage within the clan is strictly taboo. Polygamy is not practised but divorce and remarriages are common and frequent. Also the system of dowry was unknown, rather a kind of price for the bride in the form of paddy, fish, *dao,* baskets or some other articles were presented to the parents of the bride. Once this is accepted by the other end, a date for the marriage is set. This form is, however, not obligatory or considered a norm, as most marriages among the Aos was of free choice and mutual understanding. Generally the marriageable age for an individual is between fifteen to twenty-five years of age. The Aos still adhere to the traditional norms of marriage negotiation though the main ceremony and ritual is held according to Christian teachings.

Death Ceremonies

The experience of death also plays a pivotal role in Ao society, which is generally followed by elaborate rituals and ceremonies. Even prior to acceptance of the Christian faith, the Aos believed in a life after death with the two main notion of life after death, in that: a) life after death is much the same as it is on earth, and b) they need not toil in the next existence. Much the same, there are also two views regarding the spirit of a person after death: on its journey to the next world, the spirit wanders for sometime around a river called *Lungritzu,* which demarcates the land of the living and the death. During this time, if the spirit is summoned back, it returns to the deceased body, however, once the spirit crosses this river it cannot return. The other view is that, after death, the spirit on its journey is liable to be attacked by the spirits of the man or animals he had killed and so because of this fear, it does not immediately leave the house. As a sign of assurance, that it will be escorted safely on its journey, relatives of the deceased bangs on the walls and stamps on the floors. Generally a dog and a fowl are offered as part of the funerary ritual to accompany the dead man in his after-life journey. *Daos* and spears may be placed beside the corpse with the belief that the spirits may use them to ward off the spirits on the path.

Usually the corpse is taken to the cemetery during harvest time, but if the corpse is not properly dried it was disposed only during the next harvest. With the corpse dried, they are taken to the cemetery and disposed in a bamboo house like structure, raised above the ground. Personal belongings of the deceased like shawls, ornaments, baskets, disnes etc. are hung over this structure. With mass conversions to Christianity, this traditional system of corpse disposal is no longer practised by the Aos.

Dress and Ornaments

The Ao Nagas being a lover of colours and designs have their own traditional attires. The Ao men used to wear a kind of apron or loin cloth which is a small piece of cloth known to the Aos as *Langtem* in *Chungli* clan and *Angen* in *Mongsen.* This cloth is of two flaps, which is worn around the waist covering the front part and passing between the legs, which is then, fasten to the belt at the back, where a dao wooden holder is tied around the waist to carry dao. The patterns and designs of the apron differ among different clan or villages but the shape and size is almost the same. These aprons are made of plain cloth, white or dark blue in colour with cowries shells sewed on it. In some, figures of animals are painted. Another important dress code of the men is the shawl, which is composed of three pieces, the middle piece is woven on black thread with red lining, while the other two on the sides is woven on red thread with black lining on it, these three pieces of cloth is sewed together to make the shawl. The shawl is known as *Siipangsii,* which can be worn by all ordinary people.

The other type of shawl, which is broadly known as *Tsiingkotepsii,* has designs painted on a piece of cloth known as *Siimelong* and sewed in the middle of *Siipangsii.* The paintings and design on *Siimelong* differs according to the status and deeds of the wearer. The symbols painted on the cloth are human head, elephant, mithun, buffalo, tiger, hornbill, shield, spear, dao, cock, sun moon and star. *Mangkotepsii* (mangko-'enemies head', tep-'printed', and su-'shawl') is one such type of *Tsuglwtepsu* shawl, which has paintings of human head in it and can be worn by warrior only who have taken enemies head. It is also known as *Nokin lretersu,* which means 'warriors shawl'. If a man has slain a tiger, he can paint a tiger in his shawl, if a ruler he is entitled to wear the shawl with pictures of sun, moon and star painted on it. Only a person who is a warrior as well as a rich man can wear the shawl with all the symbols. Thus it is a strict rule exercised by the Aos that no common man is entitled to wear the shawl with paintings, which denotes great symbols or significance. Today these motifs and designs on the shawls have lost their significance and can be worn by any man, according to his choice.

The ornaments used by the Aos are same as those of other fellow Naga tribes. The coronate known as *Temkhu* is the traditional head dress of the Aos. The boar tusk necklace is known as *Shibu,* and the armlet known as *Khumpang.* The conch shell known as *Lakumpong* of different sizes are made into a necklace which is called as *Lakummulongzuk,* the carnelian shell necklace known as *Marzuk* is worn around the neck reaching upto the navel. The dao holder known as *Nokleptsuyu* is worn around the back to hold dao *(nok).* The leggings are known as *Jangta* the head plate as *Kupdang. Chukhu (chu-'spikes', khu-'basket')* is the casket used by the Aos during wars and head hunting for carrying spikes, which is tied around the sash known as *Chukhumangive (chukhu-'spikes* basket', *mang-'body',* ive-'hanger') (Ao, A. L. 1999: 49). The casket cannot be used without the sash. Other important attires of men are dao *(nok),* bell *(changtong),* gauntlet *(khaup),* spear *(nei)* and shield *(jung).*

The Ao women dress consists of a *Mekhala,* a type of sarong known as *Supeti* or *Teperemsu (teperem-'waist',* su-'cloth'), which is worn around the waist covering the whole heap and legs from right to left direction in the form of a skirt. *Supeti* is hand woven. Other dresses include the shawl, which is colourfully done and in different varieties. The most common and popular is the *Angtongsu.* Another important garment of the women is the bodice known as *Tukutsukresu,* which covers the upper part of the body.

The ornaments of women include hair band known as *Lemlangvi* in *Mongsen* dialect and *Kopok* in *Chungli.* This hair band is made of white thread for keeping the hair in a bun. The other type of hair band is the brass hair band known as *Yongmen.* Crystal earrings are known as *Tongpang.* Necklaces called *Azuk* are made of cornelian and shells. Bangles known as *Kisen* are made up of brass, metal and copper, *Puttes* known as *Shimpong* is worn in the leg below the knee and above the ankle.

Festivals

The most important festival of the Aos is *Moatsii, moa* meaning open space, field or streets and *tsil* means to go around. It is celebrated for six days in the first week of May every year after sowing of paddy seeds. This festival is called as *Terokni among* (six days festival) as it is celebrated for six days. *Moatsil* is celebrated by the Aos to appease the deities asking for good harvest. In the pre-Christian days, it was celebrated by seeking blessing, peace, health and prosperity from god *Lijaba.* This festival is celebrated by the Aos with great pomp, feasting, singing and dancing. On the first three days, village surroundings, wells and other village works are done; it is a preparatory time when a new fire is lit, food is prepared, water and firewood collected. The fourth day is celebrated with feastings by killing of pigs and distributing to all the villagers. Celebration begins with games played by all, especially tug of war and games of sword bean seeds etc. This continues till the next day with all the people taking part in dancing, singing and drinking. The sixth day, which is the last day of the festival, ends by cleaning the houses and washing oneself. The next day normal life returns to the village.

Nowadays *Moastsii* festival is observed for only four days with great pomp and grandeur and dancing, singing and feasting in a rather in a Christianised manner invoking the blessing of Almighty God, though some of the basic practices of *Moastsil* are still retained and enacted during the celebration.

Another important festival of the Aos is *Tsungremmong* celebrated in the month of August before the harvest. *Tsungremmong* is observed for three days and it is called as *Asemni Among* (three days Sabbath) with prayers and sacrifices offered in honour of god *Lijaba,* the creator of the earth for prosperous and good harvest and bountiful crops. This festival is also celebrated in the same manner as *Moatsii* following with cleaning of the village surroundings, village paths, wells etc and feasting, merry making, singing, music and dancing and sports and games, but it was observed with strict gennas.

Songs and Dances

One of the oldest custom and tradition of the Aos, which had survived till today even in the absence of literatures, are the songs and dances performed in different occasions. All functions and occasions are followed by singing and dancing. An occasion without songs was considered incomplete. Instruments usually do not accompany the singer, the Ao cultural songs are sung independently without instruments, which can be of eight to nine different tunes. As stated by Imchen (1993: 130) "A simple song of a few lines is a whole piece of history. There are at least 18 types of songs of different aspects of life, nature, history, politics, social and philosophy". Originally all Ao traditional songs were sung in *Mongsen* dialect but with the arrival of the missionaries and the making of *Chungli* dialect as the common language most of these traditional songs are now translated into *Chungli* dialect. Dances are an integral part of all festivals, the *Moatsii* festival dance consists of two parts; the first section usually follows body movements and showing of their finery. It is followed by a dance, which is known as fish dance *(Angii Iwzii* in *Chungli* and *Anga malu* in *Mongsen)* where the dancers move in column of four formations wheeling about in different directions.

Another important dance is the imitation of Chang dance *(Miri yari* in *Chungli* and *Mechunger tsiingsang* in *Mongsen)* only males take part in this dance. Another dance is the moon dance *(Yita Iwzii* in *Chungli* and *Lata malu* in *mongsen)* in which only females take part.

Musical Instruments

Like all other tribes of Nagas, Aos are also great lovers of music. Some of the musical instruments are: (a) Log Drum *(Tongten* or *Siingkong);* (b) Bamboo Flute *(Jemji* or *Penpa);* (c) Bamboo Mouth Organ *(Tepang Kongki);* (d) Trumpet *(Jangzil* or *Tsili);* (e) Cup Violin *(Am Kongki);* (f) Drum *(Asem* or *Aphen).*

BODY IMAGE AND HUMAN REPRODUCTION: Ao NAGA PERCEPTION

Interviews with Ao Naga respondents presented two views about body image and human reproduction. The elderly Ao

Nagas still have their traditional perceptions about human body and the reproduction system. The traditional elderly Ao Nagas associate body and reproduction to their wisdom and traditional knowledge passed on to them by their forefathers.

However, the younger generation is aware of the allopathic and scientific knowledge of body physiology, anatomy, reproduction etc. Influence of Christianity for over a century and exposure to modernisation have changed the outlook of the younger generation of Ao Nagas. They have started using modem birth control and contraceptive practices.

BIRTH CONTROL PRACTICES: CHANGING PERCEPTIONS

Ao Nagas youth are temporarily migrating to mega cities of India such as Delhi, Bombay, Pune, Kolkata, Bangalore etc. for higher education. Their exposure to modern and urban life including formal education is certainly changing their perceptions towards small family norms.

These youth have started adopting the use of condoms, oral pills, copper T and family planning operations after getting married. This is not to say that there are no traditional practices of birth control among the Ao Nagas. There is a need to conduct informal and indepth research in this area.

THE PROCESS OF DELIVERY

The T.B.A's play an important part in process of delivery. Among the Ao Nagas there are female T.B.A's who perform deliveries at home, especially in the remote village. In case of complications a woman is referred to the hospital.

IMPACT OF CHRISTIANITY AND MODERANISATION

The Ao tribe in Nagaland constitute one of the major tribal or folk communities. Such folk societies though distantly located from each other, seem to share and exhibit a typical constellation of life style features that are universally recognisable. However, societies and cultures are dynamic and subjected to change due to internal and external factors. The contemporary Ao Naga society is in flux as an outcome of rapid social change. It is nevertheless true that the processes of technological advancement, moden education, social mobility and changing occupation structure are responsible for the changes that are taking place in north-east region and in the Ao society, a fact, which cannot be ignored. The changes are the outcome of the access of varied systems resulting from contact with different cultures and ideologies. Traditionally their life was based on agriculture, hunting, fishing and gathering forest products. However the all comprehensive change was spearheaded by the Christian missionaries and the British rulers.

The traditional-religion as well as ritualistic cultural activities such as, festivals, songs, dances, birth ceremonies, marriage ceremonies and death rituals, which basically have been associated with traditional religious ideology were prohibited. Nevertheless, some of the cultural activities still persist but mixed with some elements of Christian teachings. The contact with other community also led to easier communication and access to markets which introduced and provided import of many foreign products. These introductions caused decline in the use of traditional household accessories and traditional dresses and were increasingly replaced by enamelled and polished cooking wares and western cloths. However, during important festivals and functions traditional attires are still exhibited.

Conversion of Aos to Christianity by the missionaries also led to the decline of *Ariju* (boy's dormitory) and *Zuki* (girl's dormitory) educational institutions for learning. Formal educational system was introduced by the American missionaries and the British government amongst the Aos, which in turn opened up new vistas in their mode of thinking and thus, many mission schools, government schools and colleges were founded and the masses became inclined toward new teachings and developments. The impact of western education was felt in the political, social, cultural and economic spheres. Western education further provided opportunities to seek employment in government services and also develop new business ventures. It has been observed that the generations are drawn more towards western cultures and their understanding of traditional customs and cultures are gradually fading away. The traditional roles have lost much of its glory because the social structure of the Aos has been radically transformed under the entity of Christianity. Material change takes lead over the non-material one, comparatively well off families have readily adjusted and adapted to the change situation, whereas the average ones stick to religious tradition more firmly. Therefore, it is necessary to preserve and revitalise the traditional form of culture, so that the rich Ao culture, beliefs and practices will not be forgotten.

REFERENCES

Ao, A.L. 1999. *Naga Cultural Attires and Musical Instruments.* New Delhi: Concept Publishing Company.

Ao, T. 1999. *The Ao-Naga Oral Tradition.* Baroda: Bhasha Publications.

Atsongsanger, M. 1995. *Christian Education and Social Change.* Guwahati: Christian Literature Centre.

Directorate of Economics and Statistics, Nagaland, Kohima 2002. *Statistical Hand Book of Nagaland 2001.* Kohima: Directorate of Economics and Statistics, Nagaland.

Directorate of Rural Development Nagaland, Kohima 2001. *Government of Nagaland Department of Rural Development: No. of VDBS, No. of Households, Rural Population of Recognised Villages* (As Per Census of India) in Nagaland 2001.

Imchen, P. 1993. *Ancient Ao Naga Religion and Culture.* Delhi: Har - Anand Publications.

Mills, J. P. 1926. *The Ao Nagas.* London: Macmillan and Co. Ltd.

Nagaland Post 1992. *Ancient Artifacts in Chungliyimti,* Wednesday, July 22.

Nienu, V.1974. Recent Prehistoric Discoveries in Nagaland—A Survey, *Highlanders,* Vol. II, No. I: 5-7.

9

Summary, Conclusions and Recommendations

SUMMARY

Selecting a subject like understanding tribal concepts of medicine, body image, birth control and contraceptive practices by the researchers has been due to the fact that though there are few research papers and documentations on these areas, these concepts have very little role to play in the primary health care of the tribal areas of the country, the health care and health education lobby in the tribal areas has been dominated by allopathic practitioners and paramedical workers who consider tribal beliefs and practices as supernatural and non-scientific. This has led to a vast gap between tribal beliefs and practices regarding the above topics and the perceptions of the health care providers.

As authors of the book, we have been working in the tribal areas throughout the country for the last twenty years, especially in the field of medical anthropology, ethno-medicine and tribal health. After searching literature on the topic selected we felt that there is a need to document tribal beliefs and practices on the above subject. Hence, to initiate interest among social, health and medical scientists, we took five tribes to document their belief systems. We believe that the model of documentation, the methodology adopted and the recommendations given to the researchers as well as the policy makers will certainly be of immense use in planning, implementing, monitoring and following up health care and education programmes for the tribals of India.

We strongly believe that each tribe has unique and distinct beliefs and practices regarding body image, human reproduction, birth control and contraception. Therefore, tribe specific studies all over the country and even in the other parts of the world will generate interesting data, concepts, theoretical insights, and tribe specific modules of health care and education. For research scholars in the field of social, health and medical sciences, disciplines like botany, ethno-botany, ethno-biology, biochemistry and pharmacology can also contribute to a great extent by analysing the scientific contents and practices of the tribals in the areas discussed in the book. Medical resource management models based on the traditional knowledge of tribals can be developed on scientific lines so as to help them. Thus studies of this sort can contribute in exploring scientific as well as superstitious practices among the tribals throughout the country. We firmly believe that by 2020, while India is going to become super-power in the world on one hand, the policy makers also need to think about the tribal perceptions, beliefs and practices. Though, the country is progressing in several facets at a rapid pace concurrently the tribals also must see the light of development and should be party to the super power concept.

Neglected Area

On one hand India has a tribal population of 84 million, comprising of almost 750 tribes, having distinct ethno-medical practices which have been developed on trial and error basis over centuries and are also intertwined with the cultural symbolism of every group. Hence, they are not only meaningful but also reliable from the perspective of tribal people. Another aspect about tribals having complete faith in their medical system is also related with the availability of and accessibility to the practitioners such as traditional birth attendants, shamans, herbalists, bone setters etc, anytime at any hour of the day or night.

On the other hand the health care providers which include district health officer (at the district level), medical officer (at the PHC level) and staff of the Sub-Center at the village and hamlet level fully base their health care and health education services to the tribals who totally believe in some other medical practice. This aspect has created a debate about the receptivity of the tribals to allopathic medicine, e.g. a tribal patient suffering from measles or chicken pox refuses to take a vaccine as he believes that the origin of the cause of these diseases is due to the visitation of goddesses (Devi/Baya) and hence avoid aggravating these divine beings by taking a vaccine which is not liked by the goddesses.

In the light of the above debates, it becomes important for the health care providers who have their base in science as well as the tribal medical practitioners and elites to come out with a package of health care and education which will be accepted by the tribals as there is a wide gap that has been existing since ages among the tribal and modern rational of medicine.

Based on the secondary and primary data collected, it becomes necessary at this juncture to discuss certain issues regarding tribal medicine, body image, birth control, their notions of human reproduction, contraception and the therapies used by them in this regard.

(a) Correlation of body image with therapy

Tribals have their own concepts of body image, various body systems, their functions and the elements that contribute in functioning of these systems, e.g. the Thakars believe that there is blood in the body which is moved by the air element, therefore blood circulation takes place. Similarly, other elements such as fire or heat contribute in digesting food, water and food contributes in formation of blood. Furthermore according to the Thakars, breast milk is produced from blood, e.g. their rationale regarding this statement is when a lactating mother consumes cold food such as curd, ice cream etc, she produces cold blood which further gives rise to cold breast milk, which when consumed by the newborn gives rise to cold. With regards to chilly hot food, he blood becomes hot and therefore the milk becomes hot and leads to diarrhoea and dysentery in the child. Scabies, according to the Thakars is caused when a person eats sweet foods, gives rise to sweet blood, which gives rise to micro-organisms (*kidas*) as the sweet blood invites these. This creates itchy feeling on the skin and the person scratches, in such a situation the Thakars laugh at a doctor who tells them to take bath with a soap because for them cause of scabies is internal and therefore soap has no place as a therapy. They prefer to consume bitter juice of *neem* to neutralise the sweet effect of the blood. Thereby, killing the kidas that cause itchy feeling is more important.

(b) Their scientific sense and logic in herbal, animal, mineral, mechanical as well as magico-religious therapies

Suggestion method: suggestion method is scientifically and widely used in psychology and psycho therapy. In most tribal cultures there are several such examples where the shamans and other medical practitioners use suggestion method in healing process e.g. delayed deliveries among the Thakars have examples such as putting a root of Calotropis Gigantia (Rui – a milk weed) under the neck of a pregnant woman about to deliver. *Rui* is considered to be the goddess of fertility among the Thakars; hence her divine touch psychologically suggests the bodily system to accelerate the process of delivery. Similarly, a patient possessed with evil spirit is whipped by a shaman (bhagat) five times to remove the spirit.

According to the Thakar, the concept of human body the soul of a person is situated just below the sternum and is linked with their concept of ten bodily openings (*daha darwaje*). The first opening start with eyes, ears, nose, mouth, and the fifth that is the atma – soul is situated below the sternum. A person possessed by evil spirit loses his identity and becomes an evil spirit because the spirit takes charge of his soul. Thus *bhika-dore* when possessed by evil spirit becomes *kolha-bhoot* (spirit of fox) as he loses his identity as a human being. This shaman by whipping him five times whips the soul of fox so that the evil spirit which captures his soul runs away. The concept of ten bodily openings and the place of atma in these openings is shared both by the shaman – bhika dore, the patient and the actors (Thakars), witnessing this healing ritual, by whipping him five times and harder at the fifth time, the shaman suggests that the evil spirit has left the patient.

(c) The need for scientifically analysing the medicinal resources, therapies and techniques used in tribal medicine

Medical resources such as plants, animals and minerals – the ingredients and alkaloids that are responsible for healing and accelerating the process need to be studied and analysed. Each of the resource used has its own scientific base and has its explicability when utilised by the traditional healer.

(d) Documenting tribe-wise information on medical resources which are useful in reproductive health, birth control and traditional contraception

Inter disciplinary studies that are able to document information available with each tribe of the country with regard to health practices, healing, contraception and such related aspects should be promoted. These teams should comprise of medical doctors, health and social scientists, pharmacologists, botanists and bio-chemists.

(e) Tribal practices and intellectual property rights

While analysing the ingredients of the medical resources of various tribes in the country, care should be taken legally to provide with intellectual property rights as well as financial credit to a medical practitioner or a tribe who owns the recipe.

An attempt has been made to protect the intellectual property rights of the herbalists, shamans and folk healers who have been exposed to threats of globalisation and privatization. The Government and Civil Societies working in this indigenous territory have not been adequately sensitised on these vital issues. Some multinational companies are eager to acquire the assets as well as the traditional know-how on ethno-therapy and have initiated the process of commercialising many rare medicinal herbs with their own patents. The process of globalisation has severely affected the tribals in terms of their control over productive resources and the protection of intellectual property rights of grass-root tribal innovators. There is very little scope to disseminate the indigenous knowledge among the tribal communities in their own language. NGOs working among tribal territories are not appropriately sensitised to identify.

(f) Similarities with regard to the concept of body image and contraceptive practices in the tribes should be studied so as to propose a universal model

Tribals consider their body as a natural symbol and associate it with the bodies of plants and animals. The body as a cosmic symbol, having ten different openings is associated with the ten planets in the cosmos and with the cosmic elements such as air, water, light and heat that contribute to the functioning of the body. Their concept that everything starts in the brain, is synonymous with the scientific mechanism of pituitary gland. Hence, a lot is available that can be correlated with the scientific concepts and mechanisms that are known by the modern world.

CONCLUSIONS

Secondary and primary data gathered, analysed and interpreted by the authors relate to the following conclusions:

1. Since every tribe has its distinct cultural beliefs and practices, they associate their perceptions regarding the body image, human reproduction, and birth control and contraception practices as development of indigenous culture specific practices which are different from the conceptual framework of modern medicine;

2. Over 90 per cent pf deliveries in tribal areas are conducted at home by the TBAs because there are rituals and ceremonies associated with the process of

delivery, pot delivery and naming ceremony of the child. Role of TBAs is significant as they are believed to be special having magico-religious powers by the tribals. Hence, they are key targets and trainees for training in primary health care and health education;

3. From an *etic* (outsiders) perspective there are several beliefs and practices which do not have scientific rationale and hence are superstitious and harmful in nature;
4. The fact that these practices have been a part and parcel of tribal ethno-medical beliefs and practices for ages, certainly show some scientific rationale especially when it comes to therapies and natural medical resources which are used by the tribals;
5. Though the perceptions about body image and human reproduction come across as illogical and non-scientific, the studies by social and medical scientist reveal that some beliefs and practices certainly correlate with and have connectivity with the scientific base available in modern medicine;
6. Medical and health scientists have tremendous scope in fortifying this conclusion.

RECOMMENDATIONS

Given the above background, we feel that the policy makers in the field of tribal development and health care including national and international organisations working in the tribal areas should reflect on the recommendations given below in the interest of the tribals:

1. Format for research scholars, health, medical and social scientists for studying body image and traditional contraception

We feel that since the tribal population and number of groups in the country are quite high and each tribe has its unique cultural beliefs and practice regarding the topic discussed in the book; hence we feel that an outline of broad areas to study this topic could help the researchers in understanding the phenomena.

Areas of Studies

- Background of the tribe
- Brief account of socio-cultural aspects
- Ethno-medical systems – body image, disease and illness etiology, MCH beliefs and practices, nature and role of ethno-medical practitioners, therapies which include herbal, mechanical, chemo, home remedies and magico-religious therapies.
- Ethno-anatomy and physiology
- Impact of medicine and diet on the body
- Characteristics of medicine and diet – their perceptions
- Characteristics of bodily systems
- Human reproduction process
    (a) conception
    (b) stages of fetal growth – fertilisation, formation of embryo, development of fetus, age of viability, delivery process
    (c) complications – during pregnancy, delivery, and post delivery
- Perception of differences between males and females
- Myths and ideas about conception
- Stages of pregnancies right from conception
- Perceptions regarding the growth of the fetus in the womb
- Diet during and pre-natal and post-natal period
- Perceptions regarding birth control and contraception
- Medical resources used in reproductive health and birth control

- Research tools and techniques: case studies; interview schedules; interview guides; participatory observation; photography; videography; group interviews; and pictorial diagrams by the respondents

2. Message for the policy makers, NGOs, health educators and grassroot workers

One of the key concepts in human development is 'build on what is available', considering the educational level, the economic progress, the psyche, the isolation nature, shyness of contact and the cultural beliefs and practices of the tribals regarding health it is necessary that the policy makers, NGOs, trainers and academicians understand what the tribals have and further mobilise and build on what they have, using participatory development strategies.

Further, evidence-based research for evaluating claims of traditional medicinal systems, as propagated by many, must be encouraged and initiated. They must be carried out with the active participation of the herbal practitioners possessing such knowledge bases. This would on one hand ensure that the herbal knowledge get the scientific backing that is required to establish its claims while on the other develop the inclinations of the herbal practitioners towards a more scientific basis for the utilisation of available traditional knowledge and resources.

3. Different strokes for different folks

Our study has revealed that tribals have developed culture specific beliefs and practices regarding body image, human reproduction process and birth control and hence it is necessary for policy makers to evolve tribe specific health care and health education programmes especially in the areas emphasised in this book.

4. Tribal dialect should be considered a vehicle of that culture

The role of tribal dialects is crucial in health education; hence health educators and heath care providers working for a particular tribe need to know the dialect so as to communicate the right kind of scientific message to the tribesmen. It is recommended that pada-worker, ANM and other para-medical workers working at the village and block level should belong to the tribal communities prevalent in that area.

5. Orientation of para-medical workers and providing financial incentives

It is recommended that the workers need to be trained in such a way that they are aware of both traditional and modern practices of tribal health care. Inputs by social scientists who have vast experience in tribal health and medicine as well as allopaths who have worked in the tribal areas will certainly come handy in this Financial incentives need to be extended to traditional practitioners other than the TBAs, medical practitioners such as bonesetters and herbalists, should be involved in primary health care and education programmes. These practitioners should be given financial incentives so as to provide them livelihood support.

6. Cultivation of medicinal plants

Cultivation of medicinal plants at family level and village level should be promoted by involving ashram and Zilla Parishad schools, colleges, Gram Panchayats, Self Help Groups and Community Based Organisations. Separate funding allocations need to be worked out by the state and central government. Medicinal plants continue to provide health security to millions of rural people all over the world. According to WHO estimates, over 80 per cent of people in developing countries depend on traditional medicines for their primary health needs.

Millions of rural households in India use medicinal plants in a self-help mode. Thus, for some 4-5 hundred million people, traditional medicine is the only alternative source of health care in the absence of the ailing Government run healthcare systems. They are supported by over one million traditional, village-based carriers of the herbal medicinal traditions.

7. Understand tribal systems, document it, reflect upon and protect it

Efforts are to be made to document all traditional knowledge systems as these are really vulnerable, as they are lost with the death of the persons possessing them. Tribal practitioners must be encouraged to document them on their own and they must subsequently be provided the ownership rights. Steps must be taken to protect such documents that are prepared, through appropriate and established mechanisms.

The existing indigenous knowledge systems of the tribes need to be focussed and the state should take up the responsibility in terms of protecting and promoting the intellectual property rights and status of grassroot innovators who do not have adequate access to media. Similarly, establishing appropriate legal frameworks; promoting of a research base; and further commercialising it are equally important. The Government of India has enacted a series of legislative frameworks aimed at preventing bio-piracy and protecting Intellectual Property Rights. These include the Patents Act 1970, Trade Secrets and Know-how, Geographical Indication Bills, Protection of Plant Varieties and Farmers' Rights Bill, Rights of Communities and monitoring information on patent application worldwide. The grassroot people from these tribal localities should be exposed to such legislative frameworks.

Development Organisation (DRDO) of India have experimented on the medicinal potencies of fifteen herbs such as Ashwagandha, Bramhi, and others, and have developed a herbal stress reliever for soldiers deployed in a hostile environment. This herbal stress buster is called Composite Indian Herbal Preparation (CIHP-I). It has been tested and found effective in improving the physical and mental efficiency of soldiers, especially those deployed in high altitudes and cold areas, where they are exposed to intense stress and high altitude sickness. The scope and opportunities available for promotion of such herbal drugs need to be popularised and presented to international community of researchers.

8. Role of Tribal Research Institutes

During the year 2000-2001, the Tribal Research and Training Institute, Government of Maharashtra organised a five day exhibition-cum-sale of the products prepared by the tribal medical practitioners. 40 to 50 practitioners participated in the exhibition, they were provided with travel, lodging and boarding facilities along with the honorarium. Besides this, the money from the sale of the medicine was also provided to them. This type of programme not only fetched them income and fame but also recognised and acknowledged their skills and knowledge base. It is recommended that the Tribal Research Institutes all across the country promote such schemes and programmes so as to help generate income from the traditional knowledge possessed by the tribals.

9. Directory of tribal medical practitioners

There is a need for publishing state-wise or state and tribe-wise directory of tribal medical practitioners in the country. These directories should be published by tribal research and training institutes and made available to the integrated tribal development projects as well as national and international NGOs.

10. Interaction of tribal medical practitioners with medical doctors

There is a need to provide space and opportunities to the folk healers, herbalists, and shamans, the inheritors and custodians of the great indigenous health traditions of indigenous territories, to operate clinical and counselling services that would not only be facilitated with regular medical practices but also would provide healers with the opportunity to upgrade their clinical skills in ethno-healing practices.

11. Development of health education material on best practices

It is important that the government and non-governmental organisations reinforce and involve local people and tribal practitioners and develop good and accessible health education material on best practices followed by the tribals. At this juncture, it is important to acknowledge that a lot of these practices have a scientific base and should be leveraged upon for their own development.

12. Active role of the government

The government needs to promote traditional health care system and all measures be taken for protection of vital medicinal plants, animals and minerals necessary to the full enjoyment of health of indigenous peoples. "Traditional and Alternative Medicinal Act" needs to be adopted with a view to (i) improve the quality and delivery of health care services to the indigenous and tribal peoples through the development of traditional and alternative health care and to integrate it into the national health care delivery system, and (ii) to seek a legally workable basis by which indigenous and tribal societies would own their knowledge of traditional medicine and the government would provide resources to enable the indigenous peoples to design, deliver and control such services so that they may enjoy the highest attainable standard of physical and mental health.

13. Enhanced role of international donor and research organisations

The donors through the support of research projects on the various aspects of traditional knowledge systems could play a very important role. They would be in a better position to support innovative projects and will not only help develop and but also document and validate a lot of information that is available.

14. The role of market forces

Market forces have a very crucial role to play as many of the resources used by the tribal medicinal plants used by the tribal medical practitioners are used by the pharmaceutical companies in preparing medicine at commercial scale. Hence, the pharmaceutical companies are continuously trying to extract these resources. This has threatened the tribals in many ways. A supply chain that does not threaten the existence and sustenance of the resources owned by the tribal people needs to be worked out by formulating several networks by the government and non-government sector.

Therefore, multidimensional strategies right from the involvement of policy makers, acknowledgement of the best practices, research and development in the field of tribal medicine, channelisation of effective market forces and a continuous interaction between the tribal and the other medical practitioners can be incorporated in order to preserve and sustain the rich source of information that lies hidden with our indigenous populations. It is thus important that we study and understand the scientific and logical linkages of these practices rather than destroying and discarding the same by calling it, superstitious, illogical and non-scientific.

References

1. Chaphekar L.N., 1961, *The Thakurs of Sahyadri*, Oxford University Press, Amen House, London.
2. Hughes Charles, 1968, *Ethno-medicine in Encyclopaedia of Social Sciences*, Vol. No. X, Oxford University Press, New Delhi.
3. Kakar Sudhir, 1982, Shamans: Mystics and Doctors (A Psychological Inquiry into India and its Healing Traditions) Oxford University Press, New Delhi.
4. Joshi O.P., 1992, *Marks and Meanings, Anthropology of Symbols*, B.S.A. Publishers, Jaipur.
5. Tribhuwan Robin, 1998, *Medical World of Tribals*, Discovery Publishing House, New Delhi.
6. Tribhuwan Robin and Gambhir R.D. 1995, *Ethno-medical Pathway: A Conceptual Model* in Jain N.S. and Tribhuwan Robin (eds), TRTI, Pune.
7. Jain N.S and Tribhuwan Robin, 1996, *Mirage of Health and Development*, Vidyanidhi Publishers, Pune.
8. Jain, N.S. and Tribhuwan Robin, 1995, *An Overview of Tribal Research Studies*, TRTI, Pune.
9. Tomar Y.P.S and Tribhuwan Robin, 2005, *The Mavchis of Nandurbar: A Lesser Known Tribe*, TRTI, Pune.
10. Tomar Y.P.S. and Tribhuwan Robin, 2004, *Development of Primitive Tribes in Maharashtra*, TRTI, Pune.

11. Nitcher and Nitcher, 1981, *An Anthropological Approach to Nutrition Education*, 55 Chapel Street, Newten, U.S.A.
12. Enthoven R.E. 1920, *Tribes and Castes of Central Provinces*, Oxford Press, Delhi.
13. Singh K.S, 1998, *People of India Series, The Scheduled Tribes*, Oxford University Press, New Delhi.
14. Census of India, 2001, Government of India, New Delhi.
15. Leach Edmund, *1968 Ritual in International Encyclopaedia of Social Sciences*, New York.
16. Lotz David, 1987, *Ritual in The Encyclopaedia of Religion*, Vol. 12, Mcmillan Company, New York.
17. Bhowmick, P.K, Chenchus.
18. Turner Victor, 1967, *The Forest of Symbols, Ithaca*, Cornell University Press, U.S.A.
19. Young Allan, 1982, *Anthropology of Illness and Sickness, in Annual Reviews of Anthropology*, No. 11, pp. 257-285.
20. Van Gennep, 1960, *The Rites of Passage*, Chicago University Press, Chicago, U.S.A.
21. Douglas Mary, 1966, *Purity and Danger: An Analysis of Concepts of Pollution and Taboo*, Routledge and Kegan Paul, London.
22. Munn Nancy, 1973, *Symbolism in Ritual Context, in Handbook of Social and Cultural Anthropology*, Honigman J.J. (ed.) Rand Mcnally and Company, Chicago.
23. Honigman J.J., 1959, *The World of Man*, Harper, New York, U.S.A.
24. Tribhuwan Robin, Khatri and Ganguly 1993, *Maternal and Child Health Care Beliefs and Practices of the Mavchis*, TISS, Mumbai.
25. Carneiro. P., *Breast Feeding Patterns and Locational Amenorrhoea Among the Worli Tribals: A Socio-anthropological Inquiry*, Association for Family Health and Life in India, New Delhi.
26. Kumar, D. 2007, *Prevalence of Female in Fertility and its Socio-economic Factors in Tribal Communities of Central India in Rural and Remote Health*, 7: 456 (online), Available from http://www.rrh.org.au

27. Sharma V and Sharma A, *Family Planning Practices Among Tribals of South Rajasthan*, India.

28. Behera K.K., *Ethnomedical Plants used by the Tribals of Simplipal Bio-reserve*, Orissa, Department of Agriculture, Bhubaneswar, Orissa, India.

29. Stones William R & S. Pallikadavath, Opportunities and Choices, Programme, Southampton Statistical Sciences Research Institute, U.K.

30. Saikia U.S., Steel Ross and Dasvarma, G., *Culture, Religion and Reproductive Behaviour in Two Indigeneous Communities of Northern India: A Discussion of Some Preliminary Findings.*

31. Katewa S.S, Chaudhary B.L. and Jain Anita, 2004, *Laboratory of Ethnography and Agro-stology*, Department of Botany, M.L. Sukhadia University, Udaipur, Rajasthan.

32. Rai Rajiv and Nath Vijendra, 2005 Some Lesser Known Oral Contraceptives in Folk Claims as Anti-fertility and Fertility Induced Plants in Bastar Region of Chhatisgarh, SMTFRI, Jabalpur, M.P. India.

33. Joshi P.C., *Ethno-pharmacology, Knowledge and Use of Medicine Among the Santhals of Jharkhand.*

34. Bhatnagar, S., 1985, *Infant Feeding Practices in Tribal Areas of India*, Department of Planning and Evaluation, ICMR, New Delhi.

35. Munshi Indra, *Women and Forests: A Study of Warlis of West India*, Department of Sociology, Bombay University, Mumbai.

36. Kapoor A.K. and Gautam K.K., *Fertility and Mortality Differentials Among Selected Tribal Population Groups of North-Western and Eastern India.*

37. Nath Dilip, Leonetti Dona, Steel and Matthew S., *Analysis of Birth Intervals in a Non-contracepting Indian Population: An Evolutionary Ecological Approach.*

38. Glasier Anna, 2002 Lothian Primary Care, NHS Trust and University of Edenburgh, Published on line, Scotland mail: a.glasier@ed.ac.uk.

39. Bajpai S. and Sadgopal Meera (eds), 1996 Her Healing Heritage, Chetna/LSPSS, Ahemadbad/Coimbatore, India.
40. *WHO Traditional Medicine Strategy*, Geneva, Switzerland, 2002-2005, p. 45.
41. National Draft Policy, 2004, Ministry of Tribal Affairs, Government of India, Shastri Bhavan, Rajendra Prasad Road, New Delhi.
42. Pati. R.N, *Bio-elements in Ethno-healing Practices Among Tribes of Chhattisgarh*, India, IK Foundation of India, Bhubaneswar, Orissa, India
43. The Case of Intellectual Property Rights," *Indian Journal of Agricultural Economics,* 54(3):342–69.
44. Tiwari Dinesh Kumar and Yadav Ashok, *Ethnobotanical Investigation of Some Medicinal Plants Availed by Gond Tribe of Naoradehi Wild Life Sanctuary*, Madhya Pradesh.
45. UK Selected Practice Recommendations for Contraceptive Use, Developed Through a Faculty of Family Planning and Reproductive Health Care Expert Consensus Meeting (2002), Adapted from WHO Selected Practice Recommendations for Contraceptive Use (2002).
46. Fertility, Contraception and Population Policies, Population Division ESA/P/WP.182, Department of Economic and Social Affairs, 25 April 2003, United Nations Secretariat.
47. Kumar. D, Prevalence of Female Infertility and its Socio-economic Factors in Tribal Communities of Central India, *Banaras Hindu University, Regional Medical Research Centre for Tribals (ICMR),*Jabalpur M.P, India.
48. Jennifer Johnson-Hanks , On the Modernity of Traditional Contraception: Time and the Social Context of Fertility, Department of Demography, University of California, Berkeley.

Index

T

U

V

W

❑❑❑